THE
PANIC-FREE
PREGNANCY

THE
PANIC-FREE
PREGNANCY

Michael S. Broder, M.D.

A Perigee Book

For Donna, Maya,
Noah, and Jake,
who give meaning to all my days.

A Perigee Book
Published by The Berkley Publishing Group
A division of Penguin Group (USA) Inc.
375 Hudson Street
New York, New York 10014

Perigee trade paperback edition: June 2004

Visit our website at www.penguin.com

Library of Congress Cataloging-in-Publication Data

Broder, Michael S.
The panic-free pregnancy: an OB/GYN separates fact from fiction on food, exercise, travel, pets, coffee, medications, and other concerns you have when you are expecting / Michael S. Broder.—1st Perigee ed.
        p.   cm.
Includes bibliographical references.
ISBN 0-399-52989-6
1. Pregnancy.   2. Pregnancy—Miscellanea.
3. Pregnant women—Health and hygiene.   I. Title.
RG525.B675   2004
  618.2'4—dc22   2004044209

Printed in the United States of America

Contents

Introduction

Congratulations! You're pregnant—or trying to get pregnant. Welcome to some of the best times of your life. You've probably already read, or at least thumbed through, some books on pregnancy and gotten much advice (some good, some bad) from your friends and relatives about what you should and shouldn't eat, drink, or do during your pregnancy.

If you're like most women, much of what you've heard about pregnancy is lists of things you must avoid to keep yourself and your baby safe.

In this book I've taken a close look at the evidence behind all the things pregnant women hear they should or shouldn't do during pregnancy. I've read all the studies, examined the evidence, and talked to experts. I tied together two sets of experiences: my years as a practicing obstetrician at UCLA, and my work as a researcher at RAND Health, a think tank in Santa Monica, California.

As a result, this book will help you stay safe while avoiding the excessive anxiety that plagues many new mothers-to-be. It will arm you with the best weapon available against fear: knowledge. It sorts out the things you really shouldn't do from those you needn't worry about. It's for any pregnant woman (or any woman wanting to get pregnant) who has wondered how to separate fact from opinion.

As an obstetrician, I learned which health issues worry pregnant women the most. I learned how to take care of most common (and many uncommon) pregnancy-related problems. As a researcher, I learned that there was a science to understanding which studies are good—and likely to tell you something important—and which studies are bad—and more likely to mislead. I learned that individual studies usually provide only a piece of a much larger puzzle. And I learned that sorting the good from the bad and putting individual studies in a broader context was time consuming.

Studies of pregnancy are no different from any other medical studies: That's why contradictory results are the rule, not the exception. Think about the medical studies you've heard reported over the last few years: "Butter is bad for you." "Butter is good." "Hormones will prevent heart attacks." "Hormones will give you a heart attack." It's just too hard to put it all together by yourself.

The Panic-Free Pregnancy answers the questions women ask me day after day. It explains what's safe, what's not, and why. To help you understand the reasons behind my advice, I've synthesized and explained the results of all the relevant studies. Women who read this book can take the precautions they need to take and not worry about things that don't merit it.

Pregnancy has been around for a pretty long time. And the human body, in all its wonder, has devised many ways to protect this miracle—none of which rely on getting "helpful" advice from friends, neighbors, and mothers-in-law.

Pregnancy is not a disease. It is a normal, natural part of life. There *are* some things that can help keep a mother and her baby healthy. And I'll walk through each one of them. There are some dangerous things as well (but probably fewer than you imagine) and I'll describe those as well.

In Part One, I address the questions many women have about getting and staying pregnant: Which things can affect fertility and which ones can't? What causes miscarriages and what doesn't? In Part Two, I cover the ten months of pregnancy (the typical pregnancy lasts just a week or so less than ten months from conception to delivery) and hundreds of the most common questions women have about what's safe and what's not. Part Three covers labor and delivery, breast-feeding, and the postpartum period. Reading this book will help you make it through your pregnancy armed with the best possible information. Remember: Knowledge is power.

PART 1

Before Pregnancy Begins

1 Getting There Is Half the Fun:

How to Improve Your Chances of Becoming Pregnant

"Sex between a man and a woman can be absolutely beautiful—provided you get between the right man and the right woman."—Woody Allen

"If sex is such a natural phenomenon, how come there are so many books on how to do it?"—Bette Midler

Even before they stop using birth control, many couples have questions about pregnancy. Getting pregnant is just about the most natural thing in the world, so natural that it usually takes powerful pills to stop it from happening. Nonetheless, for some couples, getting pregnant isn't so simple. They may spend a year or more trying to get pregnant. These couples may wonder why things aren't working as they do "for everyone else," or about things that might speed up the process. Even couples who don't have fertility problems have questions about what they should or shouldn't be doing while they try to get pregnant. This chapter addresses the questions couples ask during the months leading up to pregnancy and explores some of the myths about what does and doesn't work to improve fertility.

Q: *Should I stop drinking alcohol while I'm trying to get pregnant?*

A: If your goal is to get pregnant as rapidly as possible, then stop drinking alcohol. However, if you are willing to wait one or two more months to get pregnant, then you can keep drinking in moderation. Your husband's alcohol consumption probably makes no difference.

Drinking more than two drinks a day while pregnant can cause birth defects. So, many people think they should stop completely before trying to get pregnant. But drinking alcohol *before* you get pregnant *does not* increase the risk of birth defects. Your body can eliminate alcohol so rapidly that no detectable alcohol remains in your bloodstream a few hours after you have a drink. If there's no alcohol in your blood, there's no alcohol to hurt your pregnancy.

Women who drink may take a bit longer to get pregnant. It may be that alcohol interferes with fertilization or with implantation of the fertilized egg into the uterus. Fertility seems to be reduced the most if you drink after ovulation.

Drinking fewer than five drinks a week after ovulation has a very tiny effect on fertility, while drinking greater than five drinks has a slightly higher effect. Even drinking more than five drinks a week only reduces fertility by about ten percent, and it does not matter whether the alcohol is wine, beer, or hard liquor. A ten-percent reduction in fertility can be thought of like this: If 100 women who don't drink try to get pregnant starting on January 1, about eighty will be pregnant by December 31. If another hundred women who are trying to get pregnant each had ten drinks a week, only about seventy-two would be pregnant by the end of the year.

Drinking during pregnancy is covered in a later section, but you should know that drinking more than two drinks a day during pregnancy increases the risk of birth defects. If you drink more than this before you know you're pregnant, don't panic: the risk that you've done your body any harm is so small it's hard to measure. In the early part of pregnancy, the embryo is floating free in the uterus—it has not yet *implanted* in the uterine wall. Things in your bloodstream have a much harder time reaching the embryo at this stage, compared with after the embryo implants. There is no placenta before implantation, so chances are that none of the alcohol you drank got to the baby.

Q: *Should I cut out coffee while I'm trying to get pregnant? What about tea and cola drinks?*

A: There is no reason to stop drinking coffee, tea, or other caffeine-containing beverages while you're trying to get pregnant. Many scientists have looked for a link between the use of caffeinated drinks and decreased fertility and they haven't found it. In fact, researchers at Kaiser Permanente in Northern California studied 200 women and found that drinking a cup and a half of tea a day *increased* the odds of getting pregnant. Don't start drinking tea in order to get pregnant (this was only a small study), but this study does show that caffeine probably has nothing to do with the ability to conceive.

There does appear to be a moderate link between heavy caffeine use (that is, more than five cups a day) and early spontaneous abortion. You can cut back on coffee *after* you get pregnant if you currently drink more than five cups a day. If you don't drink more than five cups a day, then cutting back (even after you get pregnant) isn't necessary.

This is one of those issues where I find people have trouble believing the evidence. There have been so many news reports about caffeine that it may seem unbelievable that it's not dangerous to pregnant women. Those reports don't give a clear picture of what's going on. Heavy caffeine use *does* slightly increase the risk of spontaneous abortion, so many people incorrectly assume this means even low levels of caffeine use are dangerous. The truth is that all of the published scientific studies looking at low levels of caffeine intake have found absolutely no relationship between low caffeine intake and pregnancy loss. For many substances that women have questions about in pregnancy, there are no studies that have determined if they are or aren't dangerous. But we can truly say there is positive evidence that small amounts of caffeine are not harmful to pregnancy.

Q: *Should my husband quite drinking coffee while we're trying to get pregnant?*

A: There is no reason for your husband to stop drinking coffee. There was one published report stating that caffeine seemed to increase the movement of sperm, but there is no report on whether this increases or decreases the likelihood of pregnancy.

Q: *Are there any special diets that will increase my chances of getting pregnant?*

A: No diet is going to help you get pregnant. Pregnancy is one of the most important functions of the human body and it's possible to get pregnant with the worst diet that you can imagine. This is not to say that you shouldn't try to improve your diet, because you certainly should. You should improve your diet because it will make you live longer, make you feel better, and possibly reduce the risk of birth defects in your baby, but a special diet won't help you get pregnant. (See **Improving Your Odds of Getting Pregnant** at the end of this chapter for some advice on how to do that.) Having adequate folic acid in your diet can help to reduce the risk of spinal cord defects in your baby, but it won't help you get pregnant. To reduce your baby's risk of spinal cord defects, begin taking a folic acid supplement of 400 mcg/day as soon as you stop using birth control (see Chapter 4).

Q: *Is there a good body weight I should be at before I try to get pregnant?*

A: If your weight is relatively normal, then you don't have to do anything. But some women probably should gain or lose weight before they try to get pregnant. For example, if you are extremely athletic and have a very low body-fat level, you may not be ovulating regularly. Without ovulating, you won't be able to get pregnant. In today's sedentary society, this is a problem for only a very small group of women.

Obese women may have more trouble getting pregnant. Certainly, being overweight is not good for your health in the long run. It's less clear that losing weight will help you get pregnant right away. Some obese women have a condition called *polycystic ovary syndrome* (PCOS).

PCOS itself seems to cause both reduced fertility and increased weight. So, in women with PCOS, losing weight will not necessarily improve fertility. Of course, efforts to increase your physical fitness and achieve a normal body weight can only be good for you in the long term.

Women who have proven infertility—that is, have spent more than a year trying to get pregnant without success—and who are obese, may benefit from a weight-loss program. A study of obese, infertile women showed that weight loss did increase the chances of a successful pregnancy. Remember, however, that most obese women *aren't* infertile and studies of infertile women can't be applied to the general population.

Q: *Is it true that if I hold my legs in the air after sex, I'm more likely to get pregnant?*

A: Absolutely not. If it helps you relax after sex to put your feet in the air, then by all means do it, otherwise don't bother. It's about as effective a way of getting pregnant as jumping up and down after sex is in *preventing* pregnancy. The sperm and egg are brought together by a complicated series of processes in the body. The uterus contracts and draws the sperm inside it. The fallopian tubes have small, hair-like structures inside them that help wave the egg down the tube in order to meet the sperm. The process is actively managed by your body at a microscopic level. The position of your legs, hips, abdomen, or head have nothing to do with it. If human reproduction required calisthenics like this in order to get pregnant, our species would be doomed.

Q: *How good are home pregnancy kits?*

A: If you believe the advertising hype, you would think they are perfect, but they're not. Independent tests show that for every four women who use these tests and are pregnant, one will get a test result saying she is *not*. Similarly, for every four women who use the test and aren't pregnant, one will have a test saying she *is*.

The lack of accuracy of these kits isn't entirely based on the way the women use them either. In about ten percent of pregnancies, the pregnancy will not yet have implanted in the uterine wall when the first day of the next period rolls around. These kits test for *human chorionic gonadotropin* (HCG). Unless the pregnancy is implanted in the uterine wall, there's no way for the HCG it's producing to get into the bloodstream. As a result, in at least ten percent of women, the test won't be positive on the first day of a missed period.

Add in the number of women who make mistakes, and problems in the production and manufacture of the kits, and you end up with one in four test results being wrong. You should always confirm these home tests either by repeating it several weeks later or seeing your doctor.

Q: *Do I need an ovulation kit?*

A: Marketers of home ovulation kits have done a wonderful job of convincing women that they need these kits to get pregnant, but if human beings really needed ovulation predictor kits to get pregnant, we would have died out millennia ago. Amazingly enough, there is not a shred of evidence that ovulation kits improve the odds of pregnancy. Birth control pills produced the sexual revolution because it's hard *not* to get pregnant. Pregnancy is what normally happens to couples who have sex, and in most cases it's not something that needs help from medical science. If you needed a kit to get pregnant, birth control pills would not be necessary; you'd just stop using the kit. Some couples try to *avoid* pregnancy by timing their cycles, but anyone who has done this can tell you it only works if done extraordinarily carefully and in conjunction with other techniques, like checking cervical mucus. For women who've tried to get pregnant for a year or more and can't do it, timing intercourse, used along with more invasive fertility treatments, might be important. For the vast majority of women, however, timing intercourse with an ovulation predictor kit not only fails to improve the chances of pregnancy, it probably decreases it (see below).

Q: *How can timing intercourse decrease the odds of getting pregnant?*

A: Fertility experts agree that the odds of getting pregnant drop dramatically after ovulation. That is, to get pregnant you must have sex

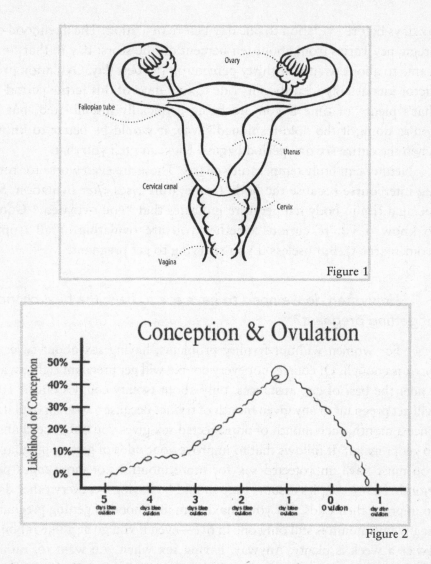

Figure 1

Figure 2

before you ovulate: The sperm must be present in the uterus or fallopian tubes when the egg is released in order for conception to occur. If you wait for ovulation, then the key moment has passed. As Dr. Joseph Stanford from the University of Utah showed in a 2002 article in *Obstetrics & Gynecology*, most techniques for checking ovulation (menstrual calendar, basal body temperature chart, ovulation predictor kit) identify ovulation best *after* it has occurred. And having intercourse after ovulation is during the time *least* likely to result in pregnancy.

You are most likely to get pregnant if you have sex some time between six days before ovulation to one day before ovulation. The likelihood of pregnancy varies from about ten percent on the worst day in that time frame to about twenty or thirty percent on the best day. Ovulation predictor kits usually identify only one to two days of this fertile period—that's plenty of time if you are being artificially inseminated, but if you're doing it the "old-fashioned" way, it would be better to know when the entire six-day period begins. Kits can't tell you that.

Neither can body temperature charts. These are even worse for timing intercourse because the body temperature rises *after* ovulation. So seeing a rise in body temperature indicates that "you ovulated." Good to know if you're curious whether you are ovulating at all (some women aren't). But useless if you're trying to get pregnant.

Q: *How often do we need to have sex to have the best chance of getting pregnant?*

A: For women without fertility problems, having sex about twice a week is enough. Of course, not every couple will get pregnant right away. Under the best of circumstances, only about twenty couples out of 100 will get pregnant in any given month of trying. Because a woman ovulates once a month, each month of unprotected sex gives you only one chance to get pregnant. It follows that to improve your odds of getting pregnant, you must have unprotected sex for more months, not more *times* per month. Many couples assume they should be having sex every other day to improve their odds. But your maximum likelihood of getting pregnant in any one month is still only one in five—even if you go at it like rabbits. Twice a week is plenty. Anyway, having sex when you want to, rather than trying for a certain number, will make it more fun. Trying to have sex "every other day" like it's some kind of sales target takes all the fun out of it. And sex without fun hardly seems worth the effort.

Q: *I'm so stressed out about trying to get pregnant. Can that make it harder to get pregnant?*

A: Probably not, but much about the relationship between stress and pregnancy remains a mystery. Most people understand what "stress" means, but it's a difficult concept to define scientifically. And if you can't measure something scientifically, it's hard to study its effects. Despite this difficulty, many researchers have examined the relationship between stress and the ability to get pregnant. Most researchers interview people to measure their stress levels. They rate stress based on certain life events that may have recently happened (for example, getting married would rate 100 points, buying a house would get fifty points, and so on). But not all researchers use the same technique and when studies rate stress differently, it's hard to compare their results.

A second major difficulty in studying the relationship between stress and pregnancy is the "chicken and egg problem." In other words, understanding which comes first: high stress or trouble getting pregnant. Not getting pregnant could raise stress levels as much as stress levels could reduce the chance of getting pregnant.

There are no studies demonstrating that your stress will make it harder to get pregnant. There are some studies in animals showing that severe stress—unlike anything a typical woman would be going through—can cause fertility problems. The level of stress in these studies was extraordinary (like being exposed to random electric shocks). It's just too big a leap to go from these studies to saying that the stresses of everyday life will reduce your chances of getting pregnant.

Don't get stressed out that stress is going to make it harder for you to get pregnant. While being under stress over the long run can be harmful, it won't interfere with getting pregnant. Except, of course, if your stress level keeps you from having sex.

Q: *How long do I need to be off the birth control pills before I start trying to get pregnant?*

A: The day you stop the pills, you can begin trying to get pregnant. You don't need to wait a specified period of time before "trying." After stopping birth control pills, women do have a *slight* delay before their normal fertility returns. And by slight, I mean these women may take several more months to get pregnant than someone who has just stopped using, say, condoms.

About half of condom or diaphragm users can get pregnant within three to six months of discontinuing their birth control method. About one-third of birth control users will be pregnant within three to six months. But two years after stopping their birth control method, the same percentage of women get pregnant, regardless of the type of birth control they were using. IUD users follow the same pattern as users of birth control pills. There might be a slight lag compared to condom users, but in the end, the same number get pregnant. (Older IUDs sometimes led to infection that left women infertile. Current IUDs do not cause these infections.)

Q: *Two of my friends got pregnant in their first month of trying. How long does it usually take?*

A: Studies of couples with no preexisting fertility problems have consistently shown that only about twenty percent will get pregnant each month. That twenty percent per month figure is under ideal conditions. People tend to minimize difficulties they've had in the past. Women reporting how long it took them to get pregnant are no different. When looking back, many women simply forget the months that they tried before they actually got pregnant.

If either person has had trouble conceiving or impregnating someone in the past, then the number drops below twenty percent. If 100 normally fertile couples all begin trying to get pregnant on January 1, eighty of those couples would be pregnant by the end of the year. Those remaining twenty still wouldn't necessarily have any fertility problems. But just by bad luck, they may not have had a cycle where egg and sperm were able to connect, fertilize, and implant.

Q: *I've been trying for six months. What is wrong?*

A: Nothing. You just haven't been trying long enough. Unless you've been trying to get pregnant (and by trying, I mean unprotected intercourse at least twice a week—you'd be amazed at the people who come in to my office wondering why they can't get pregnant when one lives in New York and the other lives in Los Angeles), then you haven't been trying long enough. As I mentioned before, there is really only one op-

portunity to get pregnant every month. That is, the ovaries usually release only one egg per month (if more than one egg is released and fertilized, it can lead to fraternal twins). If it's not fertilized, it'll be another
month before you have another chance. So, the key to successfully getting pregnant is spending more months trying; not changing your diet,
lowering stress, adjusting the days of the month that you have sex, or
anything else.

If you've been trying for more than a year and you still haven't gotten pregnant, then it's time to visit your doctor. Many gynecologists
start investigating fertility problems long before this year is reached. Let
me describe a scenario so you can understand why this helps *them* but
hurts *you*. If I'm a gynecologist and see 1,000 patients a year who have
been trying for at least a year, the odds are that only thirty percent will
ever be able to get and stay pregnant. (That's about how many infertile
couples end up with children from their own eggs and sperm.) If, on the
other hand, I see 1,000 women who have only been trying to get pregnant for six months, then my "success rate" (the number of women
who deliver a term infant) will probably double or even triple. In other
words, by taking on patients who don't really have fertility problems, I
can dramatically increase my success rate.

I'm not suggesting that infertility doctors consciously treat women
who don't need it, but if doctors don't let nature take its course, they
expose women to harm (use of drugs to increase fertility, surgical treatments for infertility, or simply the stress of investigating fertility problems) without really increasing these women's chances of getting pregnant.
Do yourself a favor: Spend a full year having regular, unprotected sex
before you see your doctor to investigate fertility problems.

Q: *I keep hearing that my age affects how easy it is to get pregnant. What about my partner's age?*

A: The father's age affects pregnancy rates, but not as dramatically as
the mother's. Men over twenty-five are slightly less likely to impregnate
their partners in the first six to twelve months of trying. But it appears
that over the long run, these men are just as likely to be able to achieve
a normal pregnancy. Male fertility does not drop dramatically with age.

For example, men over forty are only a little less likely to get their partner pregnant within twelve months compared with men between twenty-five and forty. No one really understands why the woman's age matters so much more than the man's. But it does, as I explain in more detail below.

Q: *How much harder is it for a women to get pregnant at age thirty-five than thirty? Or forty than thirty-five?*

A: The answer really depends on the woman. Most of the information about age-related changes in fertility comes from studying women attending infertility clinics. Women who go to infertility clinics usually have been unable to get pregnant for at least two years. In many cases, they've been trying for more than five years. Information learned by observing this group of women probably doesn't apply to women who have not been trying for very long. Women getting fertility treatments already have worse fertility than the general population, so using their results to try to predict how easy it will be for other women to get pregnant is misleading.

Unfortunately, no one has published any information about "normal" women. So, we have to use what we have. Clearly, fertility declines in both men and women as they age, although it declines faster in women. By menopause, *no* woman can get pregnant without some serious high-tech intervention. If we call normal fertility "100 percent fertility," then a woman at menopause has "zero percent fertility." (Now, calling a young woman's fertility 100 percent is not completely accurate because in a group of 100 women randomly selected, about ten percent will have difficulty getting pregnant, but nonetheless this group has 100 percent of their normal fertility. No group is likely to have higher fertility than this.)

It appears that fertility drops subtly beginning at age thirty. Between thirty and thirty-five, the main change is in how *long* it might take to get pregnant. All other things being equal (for example, assuming you haven't had any significant health problems in the intervening years), you are nearly as likely to be able to get pregnant at age thirty-five as you are at age thirty. Perhaps your chance of getting pregnant falls by a few percent.

Between age thirty-five and forty, the drop is more dramatic. Fertility clinics keep statistics on how many of their patients have "live births." This number reflects not just the number of women who get pregnant, which is usually very high, but those who go on to deliver live-born infants. In other words, it eliminates women who get pregnant but have early miscarriages or abortions. According to Dr. Mark Sauer, Chief of Infertility at Columbia, about thirty-seven percent of women under age thirty-five attending fertility clinics have live births—much lower than the rate for most women under thirty-five. Less than ten percent of women over forty who have fertility treatments have a live birth.

Deciding how this relates to you is the tough part. If you have not been trying to get pregnant for very long, it doesn't relate at all. A forty-year-old who has never tried to get pregnant before might find it very easy to do. There's just no way to predict.

No matter what your age, your chances of getting pregnant are higher if you've had a child before. If you're forty and have no children, your chance of getting pregnant is three or four percent lower than if you have kids.

Don't make too much of these numbers. Whatever age you are, as long as you are having regular periods, there is a chance you can get pregnant. The best way to begin is by having regular intercourse. If you're not doing this, then worrying about pregnancy rates is at least one step too early.

If you are over thirty-five and you've been trying to get pregnant for six or more months, talk to your ob/gyn. After a year of unprotected sex without pregnancy, you should talk to your doctor—whatever your age.

You can maximize your chances of pregnancy by cutting down on drinking if you drink a lot, quitting smoking, and having sex twice a week. There aren't any known ways of changing your age, so don't spend too much time worrying about it.

Q: *How can I improve my chances of having a girl?*

A: Have lots of children. If you don't want a big family, then prayer is the second best method.

People have been looking for ways to choose their children's sex for thousands of years. Around 500 B.C., the Greeks hypothesized that semen coming from the right testicle produced males and thus, from the left testicle came females. In eighteenth-century Europe, some noblemen had their left testicle removed to guarantee a male heir. (Tell your husband this and watch him cringe.)

Researchers at the Center for Reproductive Medicine and Infertility at Cornell Medical Center describe two more modern groups of techniques for sex selection, but neither way works very well. The first group of techniques rely on subtle differences between sperm that carry the X and Y chromosome. As you may remember from high school biology, the sperm determines the sex of the child. An X-bearing sperm produces a girl, and a Y-bearing sperm produces a boy.

X- and Y-containing sperm differ slightly in acidity, rate of movement, and electrical charge. There are also minor differences between the longevity of X- and Y-containing sperm. Doctors have tried to exploit these differences to increase the odds of having a child of one gender or another. But high-quality research has conclusively proven that almost all of these methods are useless. For a few methods, there is no proof one way or the other, but the dubious history of the other methods suggests you shouldn't hold out much hope.

The second main group of sex-selection methods may end up being a little more reliable, but it's not ready for prime time yet. Sperm and egg are allowed to unite in the "test tube" (technically called *in vitro*). The sperm and egg join and begin to divide. Once they have reached about eight cells in size, a technician carefully removes one cell and analyzes the genetic material. This one cell can show whether the remaining cells are destined to produce a boy or girl. This method can also identify embryos that carry genes for deadly genetic problems. In this way, doctors can avoid implanting an embryo with a deadly defect in a woman having in vitro fertilization.

In other words, several pairs of sperm and egg are allowed to join in the test tube. They are all grown to the eight cell level and one cell is then removed from each embryo. Genetic analysis identifies any chromosomal abnormalities. The same analysis will tell the gender of that embryo.

This is a very high-tech technique and not without danger. It's certainly not ready to be used as a method of sex selection, even if you believe that sex selection is morally and ethically the right thing to do.

For now, stick with a big family, a healthy amount of prayer, and possible removal of one of your partner's testicles (but only if he deserves it).

Q: *How much does cigarette smoking lower my chances of getting pregnant?*

A: A lot. In one study of young women in New York, researchers at the University of Rochester School of Medicine found that the chance of getting pregnant dropped by fifty percent among cigarette smokers. Put another way, young, otherwise healthy smokers took almost two years longer to get pregnant than nonsmokers did.

Smoking kills the ciliated cells in the lungs. These cells have small hairlike structures (called *cilia*) on them that help push irritants out of the lungs. The fallopian tubes contain similar ciliated cells. These cells pull the egg into the fallopian tube and help the egg and sperm unite. Smoking might kill ciliated cells in the tubes the same way it kills the ones in the lungs. Smoking also decreases estrogen levels and may affect normal ovulation.

It's hard to know how many cigarettes you have to smoke before it hurts fertility. Some studies have found an effect with as few as half a pack a day. Smoking fewer cigarettes is undoubtedly better than smoking more cigarettes. So, if you can't quit, at least cut down. No one knows if even one cigarette a month is too many. Just one more reason why, if you smoke, quitting is the best thing you can do for your health.

Q: *I know that I should not smoke when I'm trying to get pregnant but what about my husband? Can he smoke or drink while we're trying?*

A: Smoking is bad for you and it's bad for your husband. He ought to stop smoking for many reasons, but improving your chances of getting pregnant isn't one of them. Some studies show improved sperm quality in men who quit smoking, but that doesn't mean quitting will improve your chances of getting pregnant. Remember, there are so many millions of sperm in each ejaculation that increasing the number doesn't always translate into a higher pregnancy rate. But because smoking is such a harmful habit, encouraging him to quit is a very good idea.

For drinking, the data are even weaker. Not only is there no known effect of a man's alcohol consumption on his ability to impregnate his partner, there isn't even evidence linking it to reduced sperm or semen quality. Unfortunately, this means that while there is a good medical argument for women to limit drinking in order to improve their chance of getting pregnant, there is no reason (at least no medical reason) to have the male partner do the same.

Q: *Should I stop taking Prozac while I'm trying to get pregnant?*

A: Probably not. If you get depressed, you won't want to have sex. And sex is usually necessary for pregnancy. Some women have difficulty having orgasms while on Prozac, but it doesn't lower fertility. If you are having difficulty getting pregnant (trying to get pregnant for more than one year without success), then you should talk to your ob/gyn. But Prozac is probably not the cause.

Q: *I took acid (LSD) in college and I heard it can cause genetic damage in my baby. Is there any special test I can take to make sure I'll be okay before I get pregnant?*

A: Links between LSD use and genetic abnormalities in a fetus have not been substantiated. Initially, people thought that women who had taken LSD had more babies with major birth defects, but most of these women had taken other drugs as well, making it impossible to tell what effect the LSD itself had.

In any case, it's water under the bridge. You did what you did and now you're trying to get pregnant. Take good care of yourself during the months leading up to and including your pregnancy, but don't be overly concerned about things you did in the past. You cannot test for that kind of genetic damage anyway. You would need a test for random damage in individual chromosomes and as of 2004, no such test exists.

Amniocentesis and chorionic villus sampling (CVS) can be used to look for certain chromosome problems, but these tests only count the number of chromosomes and verify that the baby has two of each of the twenty-three human chromosomes. They can't identify damage *within* one of these chromosomes. Babies with Down's syndrome (trisomy 21) have three copies instead of the normal two copies of chromosome 21. Since trisomy 21 results from having the wrong number of chromosomes, it can be identified with amniocentesis or CVS. However, in most cases, conditions caused by problems *within* a particular chromosome cannot be identified prenatally. For example, if a baby has the proper number (two copies) of chromosome 21 but these chromosomes are abnormal, neither amniocentesis nor CVS will identify a problem.

Q: *I'm turning thirty-five during my pregnancy. Do I need an amnio?*

A: It's really impossible to say. Having genetic testing is a judgment call—only you and your partner can make the decision. Arbitrary state-

Normal Genetics

Chromosomes are the bits of genetic material that carry all the information needed to make a baby. Each cell in the body (except sperm and egg) has forty-six chromosomes; half come from the mother and half from the father. Eggs and sperm have only twenty-three chromosomes. When one sperm and one egg unite, the forty-six chromosomes carry all the instructions needed to make a baby. These forty-six chromosomes each contain thousands of genes. A gene is a portion of a chromosome that carries a specific instruction. For example, some people carry a gene that gives them blue eyes; others carry a gene for brown eyes.

Each gene is then made up of a specific order or "sequence" of amino acids. Some people call these amino acids the "building blocks" of life. The order of these amino acids in your genes tells all of your body's cells what to make and when to make it.

Genetic Problems

"Genetic problems" can mean problems with specific genes or with entire chromosomes. People with a defect in a gene called "HEX A" develop Tay-Sachs disease—a genetic problem most common in Jews from Eastern Europe. These people have the right number of chromosomes, but one gene (on chromosome 15) doesn't work properly.

Problems can also happen if an entire chromosome is missing or duplicated. Trisomy 21 ("Down's syndrome") results when the fetus gets three copies of chromosome 21. Instead of one from each parent, the fetus somehow gets an extra copy. Having three of the same chromosome causes changes in the baby's physical and mental development.

ments like "women under thirty-five don't need such testing, but women over thirty-five do," don't make sense.

Amniocentesis involves putting a thin needle through the skin, into the uterus, then taking out a small amount of amniotic fluid. Technicians then find cells in the fluid that came from the baby's skin. The cells are left to grow for a week or two, and the chromosomes in each cell are counted.

Because amniocentesis can sometimes cause miscarriage, doctors didn't want to recommend it to everyone. If every woman had amnio, then obstetricians estimate that one in 300 genetically normal babies would be lost as a result of the test.

As women age, their risk of having a baby with chromosomal problems increase. At age twenty, about one in 500 women has a baby with an abnormal number of chromosomes. At age thirty-five, the risk is one in 200. At age forty, the number increases to about one in 60.

At thirty-five, the risk of losing a normal baby as a result of amnio is close to the chance of finding an abnormal one. That's one main reason for the "age thirty-five" cut-off. But does that make sense? At age thirty-five, there is a 99.97 percent chance that your baby will not have a chromosomal abnormality. To some people a one-in-300 risk of losing a pregnancy is way too high given these odds. Every couple might weigh these risks differently.

The real question to ask yourself isn't "how old will I be when I deliver?" but "am I willing to trade a small risk of miscarriage for more knowledge about my baby's chromosomes?" A much tougher question to answer, but the important ones usually are.

Q: *What is CVS?*

A: CVS, or chorionic villus sampling, is another test that can be used to count chromosomes.

Its main advantage over amniocentesis is that the results from CVS are often available sooner than are the results from amnio. CVS, routinely performed at ten or eleven weeks of pregnancy, can give an answer before amniocentesis (usually done at sixteen to eighteen weeks). The main disadvantages are that CVS may present a slightly higher risk to the baby than does amnio, and it also fails to give a definitive answer more often than does amniocentesis.

Like amnio, CVS only counts chromosomes. It can determine whether a baby will have Down's syndrome (in which there are three, rather than two, copies of chromosome 21) or other problems related to chromosome number. It cannot give information about the function of individual genes.

Q: *My amnio came out normal, does that mean my baby will be genetically normal?*

A: Unfortunately not. Amnio—or its slightly more invasive counterpart, chorionic villus sampling (CVS)—counts chromosomes (see **Genetic Problems**). They can determine if the baby carries the correct number of chromosomes, and that's all.

Even if all the chromosomes are present and accounted for, one gene on a particular chromosome might not function properly. And amnio and CVS won't tell you anything about those problems. For some diseases, like Tay-Sachs and cystic fibrosis, tests exist that screen for problems with specific genes, but there is no "general" test "to make sure the baby's okay."

Improving Your Odds of Getting Pregnant

- Quit smoking!
- Have sex when you feel like it.
- Don't worry if you're not having sex at the time of the month that you think is your "most fertile time." Twice a week is plenty.
- Don't drink more than five alcoholic drinks a week (particularly in the weeks after ovulation).
- Take your time. You only have one chance to get pregnant each month, and it often takes more than ten to twelve months to get pregnant.
- Don't buy ovulation kits.
- Don't worry about your poor diet or how many lattes you drink.

Q: *Why not have all the tests? Won't I be assured that everything will be fine then?*

A: No, you won't. As someone wiser than me once said, "life is risk." After an amnio, an ultrasound, and all the existing genetic tests, you will know more than when you started. But you won't know if your baby will have some genetic problem for which no test exists. You won't know whether he will develop asthma, juvenile diabetes, or cancer. Genetic testing can tell you some things, but it can't eliminate all risks. Talking to a genetic counselor may also help you understand your specific risks, which may vary depending on your family history or ethnic background. (For help finding a genetic counselor, talk to your provider or see the **Resources** section.) Having such testing may be a fine idea. But going into the testing armed with the knowledge of what they can and can't do—and the risks involved—can help you make better decisions.

2 When Things Don't Go as Planned:

Managing Early Pregnancy Loss

> "Everyone can master a grief but he that has it."
> —William Shakespeare

Miscarriage, even in the very early stages, may be one of the most traumatic things couples have to cope with while trying to get pregnant. Many women don't like talking about their miscarriages. As a result, most women trying to get pregnant don't realize that losing an early pregnancy is as common as having a successful one. More than half of pregnancies detected at the very early stages will be lost. These losses generally don't mean anything about your ability to get and stay pregnant in the future, but that doesn't make them any less painful. This chapter provides answers to the most frequent questions about early pregnancy loss—what things may increase the chance of miscarriage, and what kinds of things you don't need to worry about. The answers will help you understand the risk (or lack of risk) of drinking coffee, getting a chest X-ray, exercising, or dyeing your hair.

Q: *I started spotting at five weeks. Does this mean I'm losing my baby?*

A: No. Definitely not. If you ask new moms if they had bleeding before they were ten weeks pregnant, about one in three would say yes. A small amount of bleeding early in pregnancy is quite normal. Many women experience "implantation spotting" at the time of their expected period. Doctors think this bleeding comes from hormone changes when the embryo that has been floating in the uterus finally puts down roots and attaches to the uterine wall. Other women have spotting later on. Regardless of the timing, a small amount of spotting or bleeding does not indicate a problem with your pregnancy.

These symptoms occur for a variety of reasons. The cervix becomes more engorged with blood during early pregnancy and the tissues of the cervix become sensitive. Intercourse, or even just rubbing of the cervix against the vagina, can cause bleeding. Fluctuations in pregnancy hormones may also cause spotting or bleeding.

In some cases, early bleeding is a warning sign of a threatened miscarriage. There's nothing to do if miscarriage is threatened, however. Most early miscarriages result from significant abnormalities with the developing fetus. Lying down, taking off work, or taking other "precautions" (like not having intercourse, not traveling, and so on) will not prevent the miscarriage.

Spotting probably means nothing. If resting will make you feel better, then by all means rest. But don't do it expecting to prevent a miscarriage.

Q: *I took birth control pills during my first month of pregnancy because I didn't know I was pregnant, then I had a miscarriage. Did the pills cause my miscarriage?*

A: No. It's very hard to cause a miscarriage by taking medications. Women accidentally take birth control pills fairly often during early pregnancy for exactly the reason it happened to you. Women will often have some spotting early in pregnancy, mistake it for a period, and continue to take their pills. While very high doses of birth control pills (six to eight pills in a day) can prevent implantation of an early pregnancy, this high-dose pill regimen only prevents pregnancy if taken in the first seventy-two hours. Lower doses of birth control pills, even taken persistently throughout early pregnancy, do not cause abortion or birth defects.

Q: *My mother had four miscarriages. Does that mean I'm going to have them too?*

A: No. There is no known relationship between your mother's pregnancy history and yours. The best predictor of whether you will have a miscarriage is whether you've had one before. Women who are trying to get pregnant for the first time or whose last pregnancy ended either in a live birth or was electively terminated have only a four to six percent chance of having a miscarriage after they think they're pregnant. Women whose last pregnancy ended in a miscarriage have a twenty-percent chance of having another miscarriage.

Q: *Is it true that coffee causes miscarriages?*

A: There is some evidence that women who drink large amounts of coffee have a slightly higher risk of spontaneous abortion than women who don't. This does not mean that all women should stop drinking coffee before they get pregnant. Women who drink fewer than three cups of coffee a day have about twenty percent fewer spontaneous abortions than do women who drink three or more cups a day. So, heavy coffee drinkers might have to spend a few more months before being able to achieve a successful pregnancy compared with non-drinkers (or those who drink small amounts).

Put another way, for every twenty to thirty women who quit drinking coffee while trying to get pregnant, there will be one less spontaneous abortion. This is a pretty small benefit to quitting coffee. So, if you *like* drinking it, don't worry about it. If you are particularly concerned, then consider cutting down to two cups or fewer a day. Smoking, on the hand, raises the miscarriage risk quite a bit more (see figure, page 26). So, if you are picking a single vice, caffeine wins easily. The effects of smoking or alcohol are exacerbated by caffeine. Caffeine increases miscarriages much more in women who drink five or more alcoholic drinks per week or who smoke than in women who don't. But if you don't drink or smoke, then a couple of cups of coffee a day are not going to hurt you.

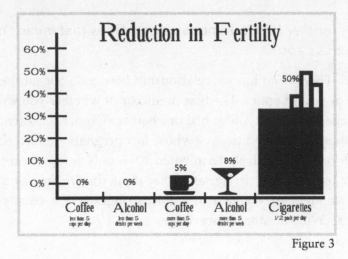

Figure 3

Q: *My hair colorist told me not to come in if I'm trying to get pregnant. Why did she say that?*

A: She said it because she saw in the newspaper or heard on the radio that hair dye causes miscarriage—but she heard wrong. Women often wonder about the effects of hair coloring, hair curling, hair bleaching, and hair straightening on miscarriage. While these procedures use different chemicals, they are similar in that the chemicals are placed on the hair and therefore may be absorbed through the scalp. Chemicals absorbed through the scalp can enter the bloodstream and *theoretically* have adverse effects on pregnancy. Several studies have found absolutely no risk involved in using hair dye while pregnant. Bleaching or straightening hair also appears to be safe.

The only study that *did* find an association between hair care and miscarriage was a twenty-five-year-old study of cosmetologists. Cosmetologists who worked more than forty hours a week, stood for more than eight hours a day, or did the greatest number of bleaches and permanents during the week had a slightly higher rate of miscarriage than did cosmetologists who did not do these things. The risk found in this study was very small to begin with, and later studies found no risk at all.

The greater the chemical exposure, the greater the risk. Cosmetologists have the greatest exposure to hair products of any group that one can imagine. Only those cosmetologists with the absolute highest exposure had even the slightest effect. Because your exposure is likely to be hundreds of times less than theirs, your risk is too small to be measured.

There is absolutely no reason to believe that hair treatments can hurt your pregnancy. There is not a single study that supports the concept that women should avoid hair dyes, permanents, or hair straightening during their pregnancy. Many obstetricians do recommend avoiding these things during pregnancy. But this position comes from "overinterpreting" the data. You can't apply the results of a study in one group with extraordinarily high exposure to all women. Furthermore, the better of the two studies of cosmetologists found no effect at all.

Incidentally, even known toxic substances—like cigarette smoke—don't cause miscarriages. Cigarette smoking clearly reduces the ability of women to *get* pregnant (by as much as fifty percent), but it doesn't cause miscarriage. Cigarette smoke is a known poison: If something this toxic doesn't cause miscarriages, it's hard to believe that hair treatments could.

Q: *I am taking medication for acne. Is it true that I'm not supposed to get pregnant while taking this?*

A: Most acne medications are not dangerous during pregnancy; however, one is extremely dangerous. Accutane (also called *isotretinoin*) can cause severe birth defects in a very high proportion of women who take it during the early part of pregnancy. Accutane is an oral medication used to treat severe acne. To prevent accidental pregnancy, women should not be taking Accutane unless they are on two different forms of birth control *at the same time*.

Retin-A (*tretinoin*) is a topical gel used to treat acne. It contains the same Vitamin A derivative as Accutane but does not seem to be as dangerous during pregnancy. The topical medication, however, presents some risk of fetal problems and should not be used unless birth control is being used at the same time.

If you have used Accutane or Retin-A and find out that you're pregnant, you should consult your doctor immediately. He or she will be able to discuss your options, including prenatal testing and/or termination of your pregnancy. Ultrasound, even a very detailed one, may not be able to pick up all of the fetal problems associated with exposure to Accutane. However, if you've taken the medication and want to continue your pregnancy, you may be able to rule out some birth defects by having a high-level ultrasound early in pregnancy.

Accutane is not detectable in the blood after four to five days have passed since the last dose, but the manufacturer recommends continuing to use birth control for one full month after stopping this drug.

Q: *I've taken a pregnancy test every month for the last four months (every time my period is late more than a day) and it shows I've had two miscarriages. What should I do?*

A: Stop using pregnancy tests until you're at least two weeks past your expected period. Modern pregnancy tests are truly amazing products that were not available to physicians ten years ago. The problem with them is that they put extremely powerful biochemical tests into the hands of the consumer.

Knowledge may be power, but there's a difference between *knowledge* and *information*. A positive pregnancy test on the day after you miss a period indicates that you have the hormone *human chorionic gonadotropin* (HCG) circulating in your bloodstream. An egg and sperm uniting produces this "pregnancy hormone." Not too many years ago, the hormone was first detectable by a blood test about two weeks after a missed period. Similarly, a few years ago, ultrasound could first detect pregnancy several weeks after a missed period.

These things have both changed. Ultrasound and urine tests can now identify pregnancy as early as three to four days *before* you miss a period. That's the upside.

The downside is that the earlier you find a pregnancy, the higher the risk of miscarrying. The likelihood of having a miscarriage declines steadily after the sperm and egg unite. If you first identify a pregnancy (either by ultrasound or by testing for HCG) two weeks after your missed period, there is about a fifteen percent chance that you will spontaneously miscarry. If you use the latest technology—either the very sensitive urine pregnancy test that you can buy at the drugstore or vaginal ultrasound—you can identify the beginnings of a pregnancy almost two weeks earlier. At this early stage, more than half of pregnancies will spontaneously abort.

Except in some very specific circumstances, taking these urine pregnancy tests with every cycle or at every missed period is a mistake. Early pregnancy tests won't help you manage your pregnancy any better.

Nothing can be done to keep you from miscarrying. Early pregnancy losses almost always result from chromosomal abnormalities—a problem that can't be fixed.

Doctors use the term "chemical pregnancy" to mean there is pregnancy hormone circulating in your blood, but no identifiable embryo in your uterus. In a chemical pregnancy, no fetus ever develops. As a result, losing a chemical pregnancy is not a miscarriage.

You are more likely than not to lose a pregnancy identified on the basis of an early urine test. Having this happen repetitively does not mean that you have "recurrent pregnancy loss" or recurrent miscarriages. It just means that you're using a new technology where it doesn't truly need to be used.

I would recommend waiting two to four weeks after you've missed a period before taking a test. This will make you six to eight weeks pregnant before you test. You gain nothing by doing it earlier. Eight weeks is

Understanding "Weeks" of Pregnancy

- Doctors track pregnancy in weeks, not months. The average pregnancy lasts forty to forty-one weeks counted from the first day of the last period.
- You are two weeks pregnant the day you get pregnant—bizarre, but true, because the week count of pregnancy begins on the first day of your last period and you don't ovulate until two weeks *after* that.
- Before ultrasound and hormone tests, the last period was the best place to mark the beginning of pregnancy. Old habits die hard.
- Weeks are counted when they end. Just like birthdays, we say you are ten weeks old when your tenth week is *over*, not when it starts. (Your baby is one year old beginning on her *first* birthday, not the day she's born.)

early enough to begin proper prenatal care. In any case, you should begin taking folic acid supplements when you decide to try, because you want high enough levels in your body as soon as you get pregnant.

Q: *I've had several miscarriages. What can I do to prevent this from happening again?*

A: Probably nothing, but it depends on how many miscarriages you've had and why. As I pointed out above, the majority of pregnancies detected at the time of a missed period will end in miscarriage. Of pregnancies that have made it past eight weeks, one in six will be lost to miscarriage. These losses are just random occurrences—bad luck. They probably result from chromosomal abnormalities within the developing embryo. The body recognizes these abnormalities quickly. Rather than continuing with a pregnancy that will never produce a normal baby, the body responds by miscarrying.

Because these embryos miscarry at such an early point, they can't be easily tested to see what went wrong—they're just too small. In other words, you won't ever know what caused your miscarriage. In research studies, scientists have used complex techniques to look for causes. In most cases, chromosomal problems explain early miscarriages.

Early miscarriages are so common that unless a woman has had at least three in a row, doctors usually suggest not trying to find the cause. I have one patient who had five miscarriages in a row and then had two completely uncomplicated pregnancies. She was sure she would never be able to get pregnant. Now, she has two beautiful children.

There are some treatable conditions that make women more prone to miscarry. Diseases in the mother like diabetes or lupus may increase miscarriage risk. Recurrent miscarriages are rarely the first symptom of these condi-

Reduce Miscarriage Risk

- Don't smoke.
- Cut back on coffee to less than three cups a day.
- Avoid direct X rays to the pelvis.
- Don't do a home pregnancy test until you are at least two weeks late.
- Don't take Accutane.

tions. If you have one of these problems, you probably already know about it.

A good physical exam and routine lab tests will occasionally turn up problems in an otherwise healthy woman, so getting a checkup after a miscarriage can't hurt. One condition that doesn't cause symptoms, called *antiphospholipid antibody syndrome,* can increase the risk of miscarriage. A blood test can tell whether you have it. If you do, there are some possible treatments. You'll need to discuss the details with your doctor since it's not clear exactly how well they work.

Sometimes, although the mother and father both have normal chromosomes, the fetus continually develops the same type of chromosomal abnormality. Testing the mother and father, not the fetus, can uncover this rare condition. Chromosome tests of you and your partner are worthwhile if you've had more than three miscarriages in a row.

Immunity to your husband's sperm and hormone deficiency are sometimes mentioned as causes of recurrent miscarriage, but the scientific evidence that these things actually cause problems is very weak. Infections like toxoplasmosis, listeria, and cytomegalovirus can cause miscarriage but not recurrent problems. Drinking tap water, being exposed to pesticides, working at a computer, and being physically active do not cause recurrent miscarriages.

Perhaps most important, bed rest is not going to change whether you miscarry or not (perhaps with the possible exception of women with cervical weakness or incompetence). That is, even if you've had three or four miscarriages, lying flat on your back after you learn you're pregnant will not help. As a matter of fact, this excessive bed rest can make you sick: It weakens your muscles and increases your risk for dangerous blood clots in the legs.

The best approach to maximizing your chances for a healthy pregnancy after a miscarriage is

Don't Worry About . . .

- Bleaching your hair.
- Drinking less than three cups of coffee a day.
- Taking birth control pills by accident without knowing you're pregnant.
- Taking most prescription medications before you knew you were pregnant.

to do nothing until you have had several miscarriages in a row. This might sound like hard advice but all interventions have risks. Doing *something* is often worse than doing nothing. Most of the time, no matter how extensively they test, doctors don't find a cause for recurrent miscarriage. Going through expensive and anxiety-provoking tests with such low odds of finding anything is not worth the trouble.

If you've had at least three miscarriages, consult with your ob/gyn. He or she can guide you through the tests and studies that are most worthwhile. Keep in mind that even after three miscarriages, three-quarters of women will still be able to go on and have normal, healthy babies.

Q: *I have fibroids. Could this explain why I keep miscarrying?*

A: It's hard to be sure, but problems with the uterus may cause recurrent pregnancy loss. Many women of childbearing age have uterine fibroids. These benign muscle tumors grow in different locations within the uterus. They may sometimes interfere with normal pregnancy. Because fibroids are very common, it's impossible to tell exactly how much they contribute to recurrent pregnancy loss. If you have lost more than three pregnancies and have fibroids, particularly the kind that protrude into the cavity of the uterus, your doctor will probably recommend having them removed. (See **Resources** section for more details.)

Q: *I had two miscarriages, both in the second trimester. What can cause that?*

A: Second trimester losses are much less common than first trimester losses. If both your miscarriages happened after twelve weeks, then cervical failure might be the cause. This condition is one of the easier ones to diagnose because the miscarriage usually occurs with contractions that are very weak and not painful. Doctors treat cervical failure (sometimes called cervical incompetence) by putting a strong suture around the cervix until the baby is due. Amazingly enough, this works well enough that many women with cervical failure carry their babies *past* the due date.

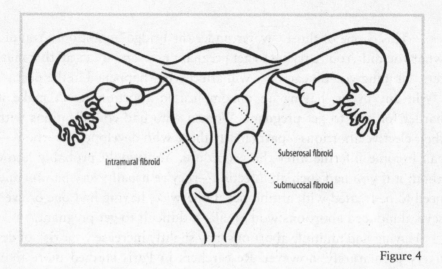

Figure 4

Q: *I just had a miscarriage and my doctor told me I should wait three months before trying to get pregnant again. Why is that?*

A: Doctors commonly tell their patients to wait three months before trying again. If you press them, they say it's to "let the uterus get back to normal." This seems like nonsense to me. Your body doesn't need help deciding when to get pregnant or not to get pregnant. If you want to get pregnant, there's no reason for you to use birth control. Let your body handle this problem by itself. If your uterus or some other part of you can't manage a pregnancy, you won't get pregnant. Doctors at the University of California at San Francisco showed that waiting to get pregnant after a miscarriage doesn't improve your odds of a good outcome.

Waiting to get pregnant after a full-term pregnancy, on the other hand, does make some sense. You can deplete your body's calcium stores and increase your risk for preterm labor and osteoporosis if you stack pregnancies one on top of the other. But an early miscarriage is a different story. Go ahead and continue to have sex when you feel like it—if you get pregnant in the first three months, great; if it takes longer, so be it.

Q: *I had an abortion when I was nineteen. Is this going to make it harder for me to get pregnant?*

A: This is one of those "water under the bridge" questions. You did what you did. You're trying to get pregnant now and that's all that matters. Nothing you do can now will affect what happened in the past.

In any event, having an uncomplicated abortion won't make it harder for you to get pregnant. Women who had complications with their elective abortions—particularly those who developed infections—can become infertile after the procedure. You would probably know about it if you had such an infection—they're usually very painful and need to be treated with antibiotics. Otherwise, having had one or even several induced abortions won't make it difficult to get pregnant.

Having had multiple abortions may slightly increase your risk of delivery prematurely, however. Researchers in Paris studied more than 12,000 women and found that the risk of preterm delivery went up by about one percent in women who had had one abortion in the past. In women who had had two or more abortions, the risk went up by about five percent.

These are not huge increases and again, this is water under the bridge. Take good care of yourself by eating well, exercising, and getting enough rest. Have sex when you feel like it, and you should have no trouble getting pregnant. If you do get pregnant, don't obsess about the risk of preterm delivery. If you begin to have contractions that are painful and closer than every twenty minutes apart, call your doctor. Most likely, everything will be fine.

Q: *Can exercise increase my risk of having a miscarriage?*

A: Absolutely not. In fact, researchers at the Columbia University School of Public Health in New York showed that exercising reduces the risk of miscarrying by almost half. That's right: Not only is exercise not bad for your pregnancy, it's good for your pregnancy!

Many doctors recommend rest for women who have had previous abortions. Women then understandably assume that resting during the early part of their pregnancy prevents problems. But think about it for a minute: If resting were required for reproduction, the human species would probably not have made it this far. There are no species known that "rest" during pregnancy. Most animals are just as active, or more active, during pregnancy as before.

Exercise increases blood flow throughout your body, helping it operate more efficiently. There is no reason why exercise would have anything but a *good* effect on pregnancy.

I can't think of any common health condition that is worsened by exercise. Even arthritis, which you might expect would be better if you were less active, is improved with exercise. If you remain active, your pregnancy will be easier. Anybody who tells you otherwise is just plain wrong.

Q: *I read in the paper that drinking tap water can cause miscarriages. Should I switch to bottled water while I'm trying to get pregnant?*

A: There isn't enough good information to allow a definitive answer. If drinking tap water does increase risk, the effect is small. There have been at least fourteen scientific studies attempting to answer the question of whether contaminants in water can affect pregnancy. As sometimes happens, the studies have conflicting results.

If there is a risk, it can't be eliminated by drinking bottled water, because there are no laws regulating many potentially hazardous substances in bottled water. In other words, while certain contaminants in tap water may increase the risk of miscarriage, there's no guarantee that bottled water will have fewer contaminants. In fact, most bottled water is just filtered water from municipal water supplies. Some municipal water supplies have high levels of contaminants and some have low levels. Bottled water per se isn't necessarily any better than tap water.

The most definitive evaluation of the effects of tap water on pregnancy was published in the journal *Environmental Health Perspectives*. Three scientists at the Agency for Toxic Substances at the Centers for Disease Control (CDC) (the CDC is a government agency devoted to examining and identifying causes of sickness in the U.S. population) examined the results of fourteen studies published over twenty years. These studies were performed in many states in the United States and in European and Asian countries. The researchers found conflicting results.

The most worrisome results showed that certain water contaminants might increase the risk of spontaneous abortion by four percent. They saw no convincing connection between water contaminants and birth defects or premature birth.

The chemicals of greatest concern are called *trihalomethanes* (THMs). Chlorine, used in most public water systems as a disinfectant, can produce THMs as a byproduct. Laws limit the maximum level of THMs, but these laws were established to keep people from getting sick from the contaminants—not to keep them from having abortions. Although the evidence is incomplete, THMs do appear to increase the risk of miscarriage slightly. Newer studies may eventually lead to tighter regulation. Water filters don't remove THMs. However, because THMs are "volatile" substances, meaning they turn rapidly into gas and escape from the water when left to stand, letting your water sit for a minute before drinking it is a good idea.

If you prefer the taste of bottled water, drink it. But it may have just as high THM levels. Also remember that chlorination of water dramatically reduces the risk of waterborne disease. If chlorine wasn't used, your risk of life-threatening illness would be much higher. And the biggest cause of babies dying is their mothers dying.

There might be some risk from tap water in some areas, but the size of the risk isn't known. The risk can probably be reduced by allowing water to stand for a minute or two after it comes from the tap. But it can't necessarily be reduced by switching to bottled water.

Q: *I had a chest X ray during the early weeks of my pregnancy, could this have led to my miscarriage?*

A: No way. According to the American College of Radiology, neither a chest X ray nor any other diagnostic procedure "results in a radiation dose that threatens the well-being of the developing embryo." After studying many thousands of women who were exposed to diagnostic X rays during pregnancy—often X rays of the pelvis or abdomen, which direct much more radiation at the uterus than do chest X rays—scientists have found no increase in the risk of miscarriage.

Scientists measure radiation in "rads," with five rads considered the minimum needed to cause fetal damage. It would take nearly 70,000 chest X rays to reach this level of exposure! Other tests besides X rays may also expose the fetus to radiation, and women may have these tests early in pregnancy—sometimes before they know they're pregnant. Not a single one of these tests, from MRI, to CT, to barium X rays, will deliver even a fraction of the radiation needed to cause a miscarriage.

Women who don't know they're pregnant and have an X ray, MRI, or CT often ask whether they should have an abortion—under the theory that the fetus may survive, but somehow be damaged by the exposure. The answer here is simple as well: No. The American Academy of Pediatrics and the American College of Radiology agree that pregnancy should not be terminated because the mother had a diagnostic X-ray examination. The level of radiation from these tests is far too low to harm the fetus.

It's not that *any* level of radiation is safe, but rather that diagnostic tests don't even come close to the danger level. Women who work with radiation sources (for example in laboratory or health care settings) can potentially face risks, so these women do need to monitor their exposure. Women with these types of jobs should be sure to discuss their overall exposure with both their doctor and their employer. For women with high exposure levels, it may be advisable to temporarily move to a role that exposes them to less radiation. There are government agencies, like the Occupational Health and Safety Administration (OSHA) and the Environmental Protection Agency (EPA) that can help address these issues (see **Resources** for more information).

3 Finding Dr. Right:

Who Should Deliver My Baby?

". . . in order to be a good doctor a man must also have a good character . . . he must love his fellow human beings in the concrete and desire their good before his own."—W.H. Auden

Not too long ago, choosing who would deliver your baby was simple; you just went to your local family doctor. Years before that, it was even easier: Your sister, cousin, or any other female relative who was on hand did it. Things have changed. In some big city hospitals, only obstetricians deliver babies, while in some small towns, a family practitioner is the only choice. But in most places, you can find a wide variety of medical and nonmedical personnel who will help with your delivery. Usually, there isn't one "best" choice for a couple; instead there are pros and cons with each type of practitioner. This chapter explains the different types of training these practitioners have and why you might want to select one type over another. It also gives advice on how to check your doctor's background and provides some resources for doing so.

Q: *Which is better, a family doctor or an obstetrician?*

A: Neither one. Quality varies more *within* a specialty than between these two specialties. In other words, there are probably just as many qualified ob/gyns as there are qualified family physicians. You can't decide what kind of doctor is best just by checking the initials after the doctor's name.

If you have a close relationship with your family doctor and he or she provides obstetric care, then continuing with this doctor might be best for you. There is a lot to be said for a close relationship and a proven ability to communicate. On the other hand, if your family doctor never or rarely delivers babies, you might be wise to look elsewhere.

As with anything, practice does make perfect. All other things being equal, a doctor who has delivered hundreds of babies will be better equipped to handle unexpected circumstances than one who has delivered twenty or thirty.

Many family physicians also deliver babies. Today's family doctor is very different from the old family doctor who had only one year of training after medical school. Nowadays, a doctor who specializes in family medicine has taken at least three years of additional training that focuses on care of the common conditions that affect people of all ages. Many family medicine specialists are extremely well qualified to deliver babies and take care of uncomplicated (and even complicated) pregnancies. In many smaller communities, family doctors are the only kind of doctors who deliver babies.

A board-certified family physician with privileges to provide obstetric care at a nearby hospital is just as likely to give you good care as is an obstetrician. Unless you have some medical condition that qualifies you as being "high risk," there is no *absolute* reason for you to go to an obstetrician. (Nor any reason to go to a doctor at all—see page 46.)

If you're pregnant with twins or triplets, or have high blood pressure, diabetes, severe asthma, or other ongoing medical problems, then an obstetrician is probably the right type of doctor for you. These specialists have more training in complicating conditions of pregnancy.

Q: *I'm embarrassed to ask my obstetrician how many babies he has delivered (he just looks so young!). How can I find out?*

A: Asking is the only way. This is your health and your baby's health we're talking about; you should not feel embarrassed to ask about your doctor's qualifications. If your doctor takes the attitude that he or she doesn't need to tell you this information, find another doctor. You can't independently confirm what your doctor tells you, but he or she is unlikely to lie. Most obstetricians and family physicians who practice obstetrics have delivered hundreds, if not thousands, of babies by the time they're reached midcareer. I had delivered several hundred babies before I finished my residency!

Rather than asking how many a doctor has delivered over the course of his or her career, you might want to ask how many he or she has delivered in the last year or two. While delivering babies may be like riding a bike, I wouldn't recommend going to a doctor who has done fewer than ten deliveries in the past year.

Once again, the lack of high-quality public information on doctors' experiences and qualifications hurts the educated consumer. It would not be too complicated for states to record the number of deliveries that individual doctors did and make this information public. Doctors would probably resist this effort but I think it's information that would be worth having.

Your best bet is to interview the various physicians that you are considering, ask them about their experience, and use that information to make a choice.

Q: *I called an obstetrician but he doesn't want to see me until I'm eight weeks pregnant. Why is that?*

A: It's because so many early pregnancies end in spontaneous miscarriage. (See Chapter Two for more detail.) If you are trying to find a doctor whose style, personality, and qualifications appeal to you, then waiting until eight weeks might be too long. You should make clear to the doctors you call that you are coming in to choose a physician, rather than to immediately start getting prenatal care. This should help get you in the door before that arbitrary eight-week limit.

In some cases, you should see a doctor even before you get pregnant. For example, if you've never been vaccinated against rubella or chicken pox, you can get these immunizations *before* you get pregnant, but not after. Also, you should start taking a folic acid supplement before you're pregnant. You and your doctor can discuss these important issues if you make a pre-pregnancy visit.

Questions You Should Ask Your Practitioner

Note: There are no right answers, but you should be comfortable with what you hear.

- Who is going to deliver my baby if you are not here? Will I meet those people during my prenatal care?
- How many of your patients' babies do you end up delivering?
- Do you do episiotomies on most of your patients?
- Are you board certified? In what specialty? (e.g., family medicine, obstetrics/gynecology)
- Have you ever had your medical license revoked or suspended?* (I wouldn't ask about lawsuits, since most obstetricians face at least one lawsuit in their careers)

*You can confirm this by checking with your state's medical board

As far as actual prenatal care goes, not making a first visit until eight weeks is fine. Your doctor probably won't suggest any critical tests or treatments before twelve weeks anyway. Experts agree that beginning prenatal care by twelve weeks is a good idea. Unless you have specific preexisting medical problems, earlier is not necessarily better.

Q: *How can I find out how many cesareans a doctor does? Do I just have to take his or her word for it?*

A: You can ask, but you have to take his or her word for it. Most doctors will happily give you a sense of how often they do cesareans, but you can't independently confirm it. Some hospitals publish their overall cesarean delivery rate, and in general, doctors practicing in the same hospital have similar practice styles. So, if a particular hospital has a thirty-percent cesarean rate, then you are more likely to end up with a cesarean section than if you go to a hospital that has a twelve-percent rate. There is a movement in health care in general toward providing more independent data about doctors' practices in a variety of fields, but this movement is in its infancy.

Along with some colleagues at the RAND Corporation, I studied how much information was available to measure what doctors and hospitals do. Our findings are saddening if you believe that more information is a good thing. For most people with most common conditions (including pregnancy), there is very little information available about individual physicians.

Many doctors oppose reporting of such specific information because it gives a skewed picture of what they do. But most people understand that these numbers aren't everything, just one more piece of the puzzle.

If your doctor does tell you his or her cesarean delivery rate, I certainly wouldn't use this as the only bit of information in making your choice. Instead, try to get a sense of how your doctor treats your questions. Does he or she rush you through them? Does he or she take the time to answer in a way you can understand?

If your doctor acts as if your questions are stupid or a waste of time to answer, then you need to look for someone else. Most of what happens during routine prenatal care is an exchange of information. You tell your doctor what's going on with you, and your doctor helps you understand the natural progress of pregnancy. A doctor with perfect technique can't help you if he or she doesn't listen to what you say.

By the same token, having a good bedside manner isn't enough either. You need a balance between skill and personality that can take some time to find.

Q: *What does board certified mean? I've been told that it's important to find a doctor who's board certified.*

A: Board certification means that your doctor has completed a certain level of education and has passed certain tests. To become a doctor, you must graduate from an accredited medical school. Most medical schools take four years to complete. Someone who has gone to medical school but has done no further training—while technically a doctor—

cannot legally practice medicine without supervision. In order to practice medicine, doctors need at least one additional year of training (the internship year). After internship, a doctor can get a medical license. A generation ago, people who did only this amount of training typically became "family doctors."

Over the last thirty years, medicine has become increasingly complex. Few practitioners these days stop at one year of additional training. Now most doctors complete a residency—two to five years of additional training—before starting practice. In obstetrics and gynecology, doctors spend three additional years after that first internship year.

To become board certified as an ob/gyn, a doctor must finish residency and go into practice for a minimum of two years. At the end of these two years, he or she must pass an oral examination with a roomful of examiners. Only upon passing this examination can an obstetrician declare himself or herself to be "board certified." In other words, a doctor can have a medical license after four years of medical school and one additional year of training. Board certification in ob/gyn takes medical school, four years of training, two years of practice, and passage of a rigorous test.

Some younger physicians advertise themselves as being "board eligible." This means the doctor has finished residency but has not yet taken the certifying examination. In general, it's better to find someone who is board certified, although a doctor right out of residency may be just as qualified as an older one.

Board certification only signifies the passage of a formal requirement. It doesn't give you any information about your doctor's judgment, bedside manner, or the quality of the care they provide.

Q: *I heard that my obstetrician was sued because a baby he delivered died, so I'm looking for someone new. How can I tell if the new obstetrician has had problems like this too?*

A: You can't. The closest you can come is by checking with the state medical board to see if there are any disciplinary actions against your doctor.

Although the situation you describe is a tragedy, it doesn't mean the doctor did something wrong. The death of a baby is the ultimate nightmare for any parent (and for any obstetrician). Even with today's modern technology, seven out of every 1,000 babies die at or shortly after birth in the United States. If a busy obstetrician delivers between 100 and 200 babies per year, then by chance alone he or she will experience at least one infant death in the course of a career. Unless you know with certainty that this baby died as a result of negligence, I wouldn't necessarily look for someone else.

The best source of information about your individual doctor will probably come from your state's medical board. A list of addresses and phone numbers for every state medical board can be found through the Federation of State Medical Boards (for contact information see the **Resources** section.) These boards investigate complaints against physicians and can revoke a doctor's license if it's warranted.

Congress also established something called the National Practitioner Data Bank in order to collect information on malpractice claims against individual physicians. Initially, it seemed like this could be a source of information for consumers. But political pressure from physicians led Congress to prevent the general public from accessing the information. Instead, the information is supposed to be used to prevent incompetent doctors from moving from one state to another without having their trail of malpractice cases follow them. In other words, the database is supposed to allow the federal government to keep closer tabs on physicians, rather than to allow individuals to obtain information about their doctor.

Q: *What's the difference between an osteopathic physician and a medical doctor?*

A: In the United States, a person can become a licensed physician in two ways: attend osteopathic medical school and become a D.O., or attend allopathic medical school and become an M.D. Osteopaths have a medical education similar to that of medical doctors, but with an additional emphasis on the role of the bones, muscles, and joints. Doctors of osteopathy incline philosophically toward a more holistic approach than do many M.D.s.

Osteopaths commonly take care of general medical problems rather than specializing in particular areas of the body as M.D.s often do. After completing osteopathy school, most D.O.s go on to do residencies just like M.D.s do. If your doctor is board certified in family medicine or obstetrics, then he or she has the basic qualifications to take good care of you. Whether he or she trained in a school of osteopathy or in a traditional medical school matters very little. The American Association of Colleges of Osteopathic Medicine (see **Resources**) has additional information on osteopathic medicine.

Q: *My obstetrician has a great bedside manner, but I don't like his partner. Should I find a different doctor?*

A: The answer really depends on how your obstetrician and his partner manage their practice. In my private practice, I delivered all my patients' babies. Although I had partners, they covered for me only in emergencies. Some practices still follow this model. In many others, one doctor might be "your doctor," but your baby will be delivered by the group member who is on call when you go into labor.

Ask your doctor how this works in his or her practice. A group practice model can work very well. It takes away the strain of constantly being on call. The downside is that you have to be comfortable with all the doctors in the group. In many groups, you will have the chance to meet each of the doctors throughout the course of your prenatal care.

If one of them rubs you the wrong way, you have several options. You can talk to your primary doctor about your interaction with his partner. He may be able to reassure you that despite your initial impression, this person is well qualified to take care of you. If you can't be reassured, you may be able to work out an arrangement where the doctor you don't like won't deliver your baby, even if you go into labor when he's on call. If these options don't work out, you might need to find another practice.

Q: *I'd like to go to a midwife to deliver my baby, but I'm afraid she wouldn't know what to do if things went wrong. How can I find a qualified one?*

A: The process of finding a good nurse midwife is similar to that for finding a good physician. Begin with word-of-mouth advice from your friends and colleagues. You can also contact the American College of Nurse Midwives (see **Resources**). For midwives, the minimum qualification should be passage of the national certification exam in nurse midwifery. There are under 6,000 nurse midwives in the country who meet this standard.

Although most of my answers in this chapter have been about physicians, there are excellent reasons to have your prenatal care and delivery managed by a nurse midwife. In the United States, nurse midwives deliver fewer than one in ten babies. But this doesn't make a midwife delivery a bad idea. A midwife delivered my first child (and I was in medical school at the time). We felt that the midwife provided excellent care. She saw my wife's pregnancy as a natural part of her life and not as a medical problem.

People would be better served if midwives delivered at least half the babies in the United States. Prenatal care is mostly about early identification of problems and teaching. Most medical care involves diagnosing problems that already exist. So, from the beginning, physician training is not ideal for providing care for uncomplicated pregnancies.

Doctors tend to see everything as a disease. Obstetricians' attitudes toward pregnancy often reflect this worldview. Midwives, on the other hand, are trained to see pregnancy and childbirth as parts of health, not illness. Midwives tend to have lower cesarean rates and fewer uses of episiotomy, and in general have very satisfied patients.

There are times when you need a doctor. Your question about when a nurse midwife needs to seek help is an excellent one. I am most comfortable recommending a midwife when that midwife works in collaborative practice with a physician or a group of physicians. Ideally, the midwife has a close relationship with at least one community ob/gyn to whom she can refer patients when problems occur. The midwife who delivered my son worked in collaboration with a group of obstetricians. If something had gone wrong, one of them was available twenty-four hours a day. Nothing did go wrong and we had very close personal care by the midwife—much more personal care than I provide to most of my patients.

Q: *What is the difference between a nurse midwife and a lay midwife?*

A: A lay midwife is someone (usually a woman) who has some experience delivering babies. That's it. There are no formal requirements or certification for lay midwifery. Lay midwives are the "shade tree mechanics" of obstetrics. You might find one who's excellent, but there's a lot of luck involved. I don't recommend entrusting your pregnancy to the care of a lay midwife. The stakes are too high.

Nurse midwives, on the other hand, have to have formal training, practical experience, and pass a certification exam. Having a certified nurse midwife care for you during your pregnancy can be an excellent choice. If you have difficulty finding one in your area, contact the American College of Nurse Midwives for help.

Q: *So what kind of provider is best, a family physician, an ob/ gyn, or a nurse midwife?*

A: None are necessarily better. Family physicians, obstetricians, and nurse midwives all may be well qualified to take care of you. Your choice of a practitioner should depend on your individual preferences and your likes or dislikes rather than on specialty.

Certainly if you have a complicated pregnancy (for example, pre-eclampsia, high blood pressure, diabetes, or you are pregnant with twins), then I would definitely recommend seeing an obstetrician. Perhaps even an obstetrician with specialized training in caring for high risk pregnancies. But if you are one of the vast majority of women who have no pregnancy complications, then any of these types of providers should be fine.

Q: *I want to find a doctor who will let me make the important decisions about my labor. What advice can you give me about finding someone like that?*

A: In truth, I'm not sure you *are* qualified to make the important decisions about your labor. I understand your desire to control the process. But remember that an obstetrician, family physician, or midwife has a vast amount of training in taking care of pregnant women and delivering their babies. If you make all the important decisions yourself, you will be missing out on the vast resources that your provider has to offer. If you really want to do it all yourself, then you can skip having a doctor at all. It's a free country. You may want to have your baby at home with just your close friends around.

Collaboration around the important decisions—shared decision making—may be the best way to approach your interaction. Collaboration should be the rule, not the exception that it often is today. I wholeheartedly support the idea that the patient must be involved in all the important decisions. Being involved means understanding what the options are, understanding why your doctor recommends what he or she does, and then making an informed decision.

The best way to see whether a doctor's style meshes with yours is to talk to him or her. You'll immediately get a sense of who is willing to

Care During Your Pregnancy

- Consider obstetricians, family physicians, and nurse midwives, as all may be qualified to deliver your baby.
- Check with your state's medical board for actions against your provider.
- Check with the specialty board to make sure that your provider is board certified.
- Ask about your provider's on-call schedule and find out who else might deliver your baby.
- Talk to friends who have gone to the same provider.
- Talk to your provider about the issues that concern you most. If you don't get a satisfactory answer, look around further.

work with you and who is not. If there are issues of particular importance to you (for example, you absolutely want to avoid an episiotomy), then bring these up and clearly state them at the beginning of your interview. Give your potential doctor or provider a chance to respond.

Your doctor may be able to give you a different understanding of the issue than you had when you walked in the door. For example, I met a woman who said that she absolutely did not want to have any electronic monitoring of the baby's heart rate during labor. After several minutes of discussion, it became clear that what she really didn't want was unnecessary interventions. While I couldn't agree to completely forego heart rate monitoring (this kind of monitoring has probably saved tens of thousands of babies), I certainly could agree with her desire not to have unnecessary interventions. We each taught each other something and came to a reasonable middle ground.

Try to establish a trusting relationship with the doctor you've chosen. Don't withhold information and don't hesitate to ask questions if you have them. Once you have established some level of trust, you will feel more comfortable letting your doctor make emergency decisions if they need to be made. Often, at the moment when things go wrong, there is no time to have discussion about all the pros and cons of the various options. It's at that moment when only a good relationship with your doctor will help you relax and trust their decisions.

PART **2**

Ten Months and Counting

4 Can I Take This?

Drugs, Vitamins, and Alternative Treatments

"The desire to take medicine is perhaps the greatest feature
which distinguishes man from animals."—William Osler

We are a society that often looks for solutions to our medical problems
in pill form. Except in pregnancy. Pregnant women take prenatal vitamins with a nearly religious fervor, and avoid all other medicines just as
religiously. Is that the right approach? It may not be. There are hundreds of medications that, if needed, can safely be taken in pregnancy.
In fact, there are fewer than two dozen medications that have any effect
at all on a developing pregnancy. Perhaps even more surprisingly, many
women may not need prenatal vitamins. This chapter addresses questions about which medications and medical treatments are and aren't
safe during pregnancy. It includes specific advice on drug treatments for
common problems like colds, headaches, and infections, and for chronic
conditions like high blood pressure, epilepsy, and diabetes.

Q: *Are prenatal vitamins necessary?*

A: For most women reading this book, probably not. Women with
reasonably healthy diets do not need vitamin supplementation. Multivitamin supplementation can help improve pregnancy outcomes in women
who have very poor nutrition. Women who eat mostly processed foods
(rather than foods closer to their raw or natural state) are more likely to

have vitamin deficiencies. Taking prenatal vitamins has become routine because they are simple to provide and because recommending them relieves your physician of having to take a nutrition history—not because they do much good.

So many women become nauseated from taking prenatal vitamins, and then feel guilty when they stop, that I've stopped prescribing them routinely. Instead, I recommend a folic acid supplement to reduce the risk of neural tube defects (see below), iron for women with chronic or preexisting anemia, and calcium supplementation for women whose diets are deficient in calcium. Most women don't need most of the vitamins and minerals in a multivitamin and the side effects can be quite bothersome.

Calcium supplements can reduce the risk of elevated blood pressure in pregnancy, particularly in women who have borderline blood pressure when they start their pregnancy. Calcium is the basic building block of bone and most American girls and women do not get enough calcium in their diets. Calcium supplements for women who eat fewer than three servings of dairy products a day are a good idea. Getting enough calcium aids long-term health but does not improve the outcome of pregnancy.

Most women don't quite believe my recommendation that they don't need to take vitamins. It has become so standard that when I don't prescribe them, many women seem to think that I have forgotten. These women tend to be highly educated and have better diets than most people, so it's rather ironic that people with the best diets are the most intent on taking vitamins.

Q: *I sometimes forget to take the folate supplement that my doctor recommended. Am I endangering my baby?*

A: Folic acid or folate supplements taken before pregnancy and during the first six weeks of pregnancy help lower the risk of certain birth defects. These defects (which are called "open neural tube defects" and include spina bifida) complicate five out of every 1,000 pregnancies in the United States. Supplementing your diet with folate during and before pregnancy will reduce this risk by half. Forgetting your pills once in a while won't matter; your risk will still be lower than if you don't take them at all.

Women who are planning pregnancy or who are less than twelve weeks pregnant should take between 400 and 800 micrograms a day of folic acid. In the United States, processed grain products (like breads and cereals) are now fortified with folic acid, but it's unclear if this fortification provides all women with their prenatal needs. As a result, I recommend that women planning pregnancy or in the first trimester take a daily 400-microgram supplement of folic acid. You should begin taking this supplement as soon as you stop using birth control, since it works best if folate levels are high enough at the time you get pregnant.

Q: *The iron my doctor prescribed makes me constipated. What will happen if I don't take it?*

A: Your constipation will go away. Unless you are severely anemic, nothing bad will happen. Iron has never been demonstrated to improve the outcome of the fetus in any way. The only reason to take it is to prevent anemia in the mother. It's true that women generally become somewhat anemic during pregnancy and iron supplements can reduce anemia. But to some extent, anemia is a normal part of pregnancy.

During pregnancy the body takes on more water, diluting the blood and producing anemia. This "gestational anemia" is not harmful. Taking iron *will* increase your blood count and reduce gestational anemia, but you won't benefit from it since gestational anemia isn't dangerous.

If you have severe anemia (not just gestational anemia), you *will* benefit by taking iron. Severe anemia causes fatigue and increases the risk that you will need a blood transfusion in the unlikely event that you have a hemorrhage at childbirth.

Certain people are at higher risk for anemia. Particularly, vegetarians may have difficulty getting enough iron because the iron in red meat is absorbed more easily than iron in other foods. Green vegetables, beans, lentils, nuts, dried fruit, and some breakfast cereals have iron in them and these can be good sources if you are a vegetarian.

Q: *When I was pregnant with my first child, my doctor told me not to take my allergy medicine, but my new doctor says it's fine. Who is right?*

A: Your new doctor. Other than vitamins, antihistamines are the most commonly used medications in early pregnancy. Diphenhydramine (Benadryl), chlorpheniramine (Chlortrimeton), and doxylamine (Unisom) are the most commonly used antihistamines in the United States. These and other antihistamines have been extensively studied during early pregnancy.

Not only are antihistamines safe, but a recent study showed that women who took them had a slightly *lower* risk of having a baby with a major malformation. Why? Antihistamines can reduce morning sickness (see Chapter 5). Women who aren't vomiting get better nutrition, and this might reduce malformations. Even when taken every day, these drugs are not harmful in any way.

During pregnancy, many women take the approach that if they can possibly live without something, then they should, because "who knows what effect it might have?" After a decade taking care of pregnant women and examining research on the effects of drugs during pregnancy, I've concluded that this approach is a mistaken one.

It's extraordinarily difficult to *prove* that something is safe. Think about this example: Somebody could walk into my office and ask me if it's safe to drink root beer during pregnancy. If I wanted to answer the question carefully, I would go to the medical library and to my computer and search for any studies examining whether root beer had any ill effect on pregnancy. I would find none.

Now what should I tell this woman? Should I tell her that there's no evidence that root beer is dangerous? Should I tell her that there's no evidence that root beer is safe? Both statements are true. Many books on pregnancy take the second approach: "Stay away from microwave ovens since they haven't been proven safe." Taken to its logical extreme, this approach would have all pregnant women confined to bed during pregnancy. But that hasn't proven to be safe either!

The bottom line is this: Pregnant women should avoid drugs, activities, or situations that have a reasonable possibility of causing harm, particularly if they don't have any benefit. Cigarettes are dangerous and have no benefit. It's a no-brainer to avoid them. Antihistamines have no known risk and have a large benefit, so there's no reason to avoid them.

Q: *I've got a terrible cold. I assume I just have to "tough it out," but is there anything that's safe to take during pregnancy?*

A: Absolutely. In fact, none of the typical over-the-counter cold remedies is dangerous during pregnancy. You can take acetaminophen (Tylenol). You can take pseudoephedrine (Sudafed). You can use nasal sprays. You can use almost any over-the-counter cough or cold remedy, including those containing guaifenesin, dextromethorphan, and many others.

Dr. Broder's "Safe in Pregnancy" Cold Remedy

1. Stay home from work.

2. Drink plenty of hot tea with lemon and honey.

3. Take 1,000 milligrams of acetaminophen (Tylenol) every four hours for aches and pains.

4. Take antihistamines if your nose is running (over-the-counter chlorpheniramine or Benadryl are best).

5. The minute you begin to feel sick, start taking zinc gluconate lozenges. Take one every two hours during the course of the illness.

6. Take echinacea after every meal.

7. Consider pseudoephedrine (Sudafed) if the antihistamine doesn't stop your runny nose.

8. Stay in bed.

9. Wait. Even the most aggressive cold treatment will only shorten your course of symptoms by a day or so, but time is on your side.

If you want to stick to the more "natural remedies," you can take vitamin C, echinacea, or zinc. Zinc gluconate has been studied in a variety of settings and while there are somewhat conflicting results, it does appear to help many people shorten the duration of their colds. There is no reason to suspect that zinc, which is a common mineral, would have any adverse effect on pregnancy.

Zinc works best if taken in lozenge form and if started as soon as symptoms begin. Typical doses are about ten to fifteen milligrams of zinc gluconate every two hours. The type of the zinc lozenge does appear to be important, so you should probably stick to zinc gluconate and skip zinc acetate or other formulations of zinc. Also, the effect might not be the same if you take zinc in a multivitamin form and not a lozenge. Unfortunately, zinc lozenges make a number of people nauseated and this problem could certainly be worse during pregnancy. Go ahead and try it, but stop if it makes you sick.

Many people use vitamin C to treat colds and this is also safe in pregnancy. Vitamin C taken when a cold begins can relieve cold symptoms a day earlier than they would have otherwise stopped. Vitamin C supplements may only work in people with a low vitamin C intake to begin with, so if you're already getting plenty of vitamin C, you might find no additional benefit from a supplement. Very high doses of vitamin C (greater than one gram a day) may increase your risk of diarrhea and kidney stones, so keep your intake below this level.

More Americans use echinacea than any other herbal medicine—most commonly to prevent and treat colds. A recent study found echinacea to be safe during pregnancy. Studies have shown that echinacea may slightly shorten the duration of a cold.

Unfortunately, herbal products are not well regulated and it is therefore difficult to know precisely what you're buying when you buy them. In 2001, Consumer Labs tested several echinacea products and eleven of twenty-five products failed the test. Specifically, for six products the labeling was so unclear the lab couldn't even determine what was supposed to be in the bottle. Four of the remaining products had inadequate levels of echinacea in the tablets, and one was contaminated with bacteria. As long as the echinacea you buy is actually what it says it is, it won't hurt you and it may help your cold go away sooner.

Dangerous Drugs in Pregnancy

- Quinine (used to treat leg cramps; also found in extremely low doses in tonic water)
- Retin-A and other vitamin A derivatives (retinoids) used to treat acne (topical medicines are safe)
- Warfarin (used to thin the blood)
- Tetracycline (stains infants' teeth—no effect on permanent teeth)
- Lithium (used to treat manic depression). The risk of problems with this drug is very low, so talk to your doctor before stopping.
- Phenytoin and valproic acid (used to treat epilepsy). Risks may be worth taking because untreated epilepsy can be even worse for the baby.
- ACE inhibitors (used to treat high blood pressure). There are safer drugs for high blood pressure.
- Blue cohosh (an herb that may cause heart problems in the fetus)

Q: *My friend gave me some herbs to help me with a headache. How can I tell if they are safe in pregnancy? (I don't want to ask my doctor because he thinks herbs are useless.)*

A: While I disagree with your doctor that herbs are useless, in this case I think you're better off with more common treatments. Tylenol is generally considered the safest medication to take for pain in pregnancy and its use by millions of women without adverse effects certainly bears this out. If you have a bad headache, I would recommend taking 1,000 milligrams of acetaminophen (Tylenol) and then wait to see what happens. There is just about zero danger to you or your pregnancy from this and it is very likely to help.

Aspirin is also safe during pregnancy. In fact, it has been used to prevent preeclampsia (a condition where the blood pressure is elevated late in pregnancy). Late in pregnancy, near your due date, it is best not to take aspirin daily because it interferes with normal blood clotting. Taking aspirin occasionally for a headache doesn't interfere with clotting.

Ibuprofen (Motrin) is also completely safe, particularly in the first two trimesters of pregnancy. If taken late in pregnancy, ibuprofen and other drugs in this class (known collectively as non-steroidal anti-inflammatory drugs or NSAIDs) may interfere with normal changes that occur in the baby's circulatory system after it's born. These risks are not just theoretical ones; they have been observed in women taking NSAIDs consistently in the third trimester. Because of these third trimester concerns, most women avoid them throughout pregnancy. Again, this is really being overcautious because these effects are only seen with daily third trimester use. If you have a splitting headache and you take ibuprofen, I guarantee that you won't be doing yourself or your baby any harm.

Q: I was prescribed antibiotics for a sinus infection. Is this safe for my baby?

A: It depends on the antibiotic, but it is probably safe. There are hundreds of different antibiotics and most have not been subjected to rigorous testing to see how they affect pregnancy, but there are some general rules. As a group, the penicillin-type antibiotics are probably the best studied. Thousands of women have taken penicillin during pregnancy and suffered no adverse effects.

Almost all antibiotics cross the placenta and can reach the fetus. But, keep in mind that most antibiotics will not affect the fetus at all. The amount of drug that reaches the fetus is very small because the placenta effectively filters most things out of the blood. Antibiotics are prescribed for a reason. If your sinus infection worsens, you could end up requiring sinus surgery. This would be worse for your baby than taking antibiotics. So, take your medicine.

The only common antibiotics that should not be used in pregnancy are tetracycline and other drugs in the tetracycline class. These drugs deposit in baby teeth and discolor them. This happens only if tetracycline is taken after about twenty weeks of pregnancy (after the halfway point in your pregnancy). Tetracycline only discolors baby teeth, not permanent teeth, so the harm isn't long lasting. On the other hand, since many other antibiotics exist, it makes sense to avoid tetracyclines during pregnancy.

Bactrim (trimethoprim/sulfamethoxazole) is the other common antibiotic that is often avoided in pregnancy. Theoretically, Bactrim taken very close to delivery can worsen the jaundice that babies sometimes de-

Safe Drugs in Pregnancy

- Diphenhydramine (Benadryl) or chlorpheniramine (Chlortrimeton) for allergies or colds.
- Pseudoephedrine (Sudafed) for runny nose.
- Saline nasal spray for congestion.
- Guaifenesin and dextromethorphan in cough medicine.
- Acetaminophen (Tylenol) for pain or aches.
- Ibuprofen (Motrin, Advil) for pain or aches (but not after twenty-six weeks unless directed by physician).
- Most antibiotics (*except* tetracycline, doxycycline, and gentamicin).
- Asthma inhalers—not just safe, these drugs are vital for asthmatic mothers.

velop after delivery. This risk is *theoretical* only, however, and there have been studies of hundreds of pregnant women who took Bactrim without ill effects. Despite this low risk, there are usually drugs that can be substituted, so Bactrim is usually avoided late in pregnancy.

Q: *I used to get acupuncture for a back problem. Can I continue to do this while I'm pregnant?*

A: Absolutely. Up to one-third of women experience significant back pain at some time during their pregnancy. Back pain can be disabling, often requires time off work, and can interfere with sleep and other normal activities. Many different things have been studied to treat back pain and acupuncture is one of the best. In one study, acupuncture was seven times more likely to relieve back pain than was physical therapy.

Acupuncture is one of the oldest forms of Chinese medicine and has been around for thousands of years. The underlying acupuncture theories don't fit traditional Western medical theories but whether or not you believe that yin, yang, and qi are real, the success of acupuncture at treating a variety of conditions and illnesses cannot be ignored. Western scientific evidence for the success of acupuncture has been emerging over the past thirty years in a variety of different conditions, including chronic pain, arthritis, headache, and nausea and vomiting of pregnancy.

Safe and Unsafe Antibiotics During Pregnancy

Generally safe	Generally Avoided
Penicillins	Tetracyclines
❑ Penicillin	❑ (may yellow baby teeth)
❑ Amoxicillin	Doxycycline
Cephalosporins	Bactrim
❑ Keflex	❑ (theoretical risk only—no
❑ Ceclor	evidence of danger)

Acupuncture is extremely safe when performed by a trained practitioner. Some doctors recommend against doing acupuncture for pregnant women because of the fear that needling the wrong points could induce labor, but a trained Oriental medical doctor can easily avoid points linked with uterine activity and focus on points related to the pain.

While acupuncture isn't a panacea, it certainly is worth continuing for your back problems and you shouldn't be afraid that it will somehow hurt your baby.

Q: *I was supposed to get my teeth cleaned but I found out I'm pregnant. Should I postpone it?*

A: You should not avoid routine dental care during pregnancy. In fact, gum disease has been linked to premature delivery, so good dental care may *help* your baby. Dental infections or gum disease need to be addressed by your dentist. Be sure to tell him or her that you are pregnant, however, so that the appropriate precautions can be taken (like shielding your abdomen with a lead apron when X rays are done).

There have been some recent concerns about using amalgam fillings in pregnant women. Dental amalgams are materials used to fill holes in teeth. Amalgams are popular because of their long safety record, their ease of placement, and their long life. However, these fillings release a small amount of mercury vapor during the course of normal activities like chewing. The scientific community doesn't agree about whether these small amounts of mercury vapor are dangerous and as a result, routine placement of amalgam fillings during pregnancy is not recommended.

The important word here is "routine." In other words, a small cavity your dentist notices during a routine exam may not need to be filled during your pregnancy. On the other hand, if you have an urgent problem or something that would worsen if left alone, you should talk to your dentist about having fillings placed even during your pregnancy.

Q: *My dentist said he couldn't do any dental X rays because I'm pregnant but my tooth is killing me. What should I do?*

A: Find another dentist. Some dentists are overly concerned about caring for pregnant women. Toothaches can happen at any time including during pregnancy and this painful situation needs to be addressed. If there's any reason to think that a dental X ray would help to determine the cause of the toothache or help decide on treatment, then it's worth having. In fact, you could have more than 1,000 dental X rays before getting enough radiation exposure to harm your fetus, and wearing a lead shield or apron over your abdomen during a dental X ray cuts your exposure even more. While there's no reason to seek out extra radiation during pregnancy, if you have a problem that might need X rays to diagnose it, then it's certainly worth doing.

A more detailed discussion of radiation occurs in chapter 4, but according to the American College of Radiology, not a single diagnostic X ray procedure exists that delivers enough radiation to threaten a developing fetus. Furthermore, radiation exposure from naturally occurring radon gas and solar radiation are ten to 100 times greater than the radiation you would receive from a single dental X ray.

Information on radiation in pregnancy comes mostly from studies of animals or studies of people exposed to large amounts of radiation: For example, people who survived the atomic bombings of Hiroshima and Nagasaki during the Second World War. In other words, very little is known about the *real* effects of low doses of radiation on pregnant women. And it is unclear whether these high-dose exposures can really be used to examine the effects of the very low doses received during typical diagnostic X-ray procedures. Using the most conservative methods of measuring risk, the U.S. Nuclear Regulatory Commission (NRC) and the Food and Drug Administration (FDA) estimate that higher doses of radiation might be expected to increase your child's lifetime risk of cancer by 0.03 percent. Compare this with the current overall lifetime expected risk of cancer of about one in three. In other words, the increased risk from radiation exposure is about one in a thousand. You may ask yourself "Why should I accept any increased risk?" The answer is: You shouldn't *unless* the risk has some potential benefit. Having gum disease or tooth decay, for example, are risky themselves (they can lead to preterm labor), so if having an X ray could help diagnose and treat your problem, there *is* some benefit. And this benefit would likely be much greater than the potential risk.

Q: *I might need gallbladder surgery; how dangerous would that be to my baby?*

A: The real question is: How dangerous is *not* having surgery? For all surgical procedures except the most minor ones, there is always a concern that surgery could cause problems. In the first trimester, fetal organs are still developing, so anesthetic drugs might have an adverse effect on development. So doctors generally recommend that surgery be done in the second trimester.

The question about whether or not to have surgery depends on weighing the risks and benefits. Certainly, if you have a condition that could be dangerous to you, then it's worth surgery. This kind of decision needs to be discussed in detail with your doctor and with the doctor who will perform the surgery. Surgery should only be done by someone who has extensive experience operating on pregnant women. You may have to travel to an academic medical center in order to find a surgeon like this, but it would be worthwhile to make the effort.

Q: *I have high blood pressure. Should I stay on my medication while I'm pregnant?*

A: You should definitely continue being followed for your high blood pressure, but depending on your medication, you may need to change to a different drug.

About one in ten women has high blood pressure (also called *hypertension*) with their pregnancy. Half have high blood pressure before getting pregnant. This is the group that's usually on medication. Doctors are still not sure of the best way to treat women with hypertension after they get pregnant.

Women who start pregnancy with high blood pressure are more likely to develop preeclampsia. Preeclampsia in turn can lead to premature delivery and other complications. Women with high blood pressure also are at higher risk of other pregnancy complications—some of which can be deadly. Rarely, these women have an abnormally rapid separation of the placenta from the uterine wall, called *abruptio placenta*. Rapid blood loss and fetal death can result if the condition is not recognized and treated quickly. High blood pressure is clearly a serious problem for a pregnant woman.

In nonpregnant women (or men for that matter), doctors treat blood pressure if it climbs above 130/90. If blood pressure remains above this level for five to ten years, the risk of heart attack and stroke increases. Pregnancy lasts less than a year, so doctors treat blood pressure elevations during pregnancy differently than at other times. During pregnancy, blood pressures of less than 200/110 don't usually need to be treated, although that's way too high a blood pressure for the long term.

If you do need treatment, safe drugs exist. Methyldopa (trade name Aldomet) can safely be used in pregnancy and has been for many years. Nifedipine (available under a variety of trade names) also appears to be safe during pregnancy. ACE inhibitors, another type of blood pressure medication, are definitely *not* safe during the second and third trimesters. Calcium channel blockers (another popular group of antihypertensive medications) also appear to be safe, although the data are much more limited.

You should talk with your doctor before making any changes in your medications.

Q: *I have epilepsy and I stopped all my medications when I found out I was pregnant. Now my doctor wants me to start again. Aren't those medications dangerous for pregnant women?*

A: Antiepilepsy medicines might be dangerous for pregnant women, but epilepsy itself may be far more dangerous. Starting or stopping medications that you take for chronic conditions should only be done after talking with a doctor. Your doctor (in this case, it should be an obstetrician with special experience in treating high-risk pregnancies) will have to weigh the risks and benefits before deciding whether you should be back on your medication. For most women with epilepsy, continuing their antiepilepsy medication is less risky than stopping it.

Epilepsy is a condition that affects fewer than one in 100 pregnant women. It causes seizures, or disorganized brain activity, at unpredictable intervals. Before deciding whether you should continue your antiepilepsy medication, your doctor will need to consider the risk of the medication and weigh it against the risk of uncontrolled seizures. Seizure can be dangerous or even deadly. If you're driving and have a seizure, the results could be catastrophic. A dead mother invariably results in a dead baby, so continuing these medicines might actually lower the risk to a baby.

The down side of antiepilepsy medications is their risk to the unborn child. Some of these medications increase the risk of fetal malformations. The difficult decision is whether this risk of malformation is greater than the risk of an uncontrolled seizure.

Because of the complexities of this decision, it should only be made by somebody with a great deal of experience. Usually, this means a specialist in maternal-fetal medicine (also called high-risk obstetrics). Neurologists (the type of doctor who usually treats epilepsy) may know quite a bit about treating epilepsy, but they usually aren't experts in the proper treatment during pregnancy.

Whatever you do, don't stop your medication. Women sometimes do this in the middle of the first trimester—after they've confirmed they're pregnant. Unfortunately, this is an example of locking the barn door after the horse has escaped. Major organ systems have already formed by ten weeks. Stopping the medication then provides little protection against the harmful effects of these drugs and exposes the mother and fetus to the risk of seizures later in pregnancy. The worst of both worlds. Your best bet is to talk about any changes in your medication with a specialist before making them.

Q: My migraines have gotten much worse during this pregnancy (they were fine with my other two pregnancies). My doctor tells me that only Tylenol is safe, but it hardly helps at all. What can I do?

A: Most women find their migraines or tension headaches improve during pregnancy, but if yours have worsened you should ignore your doctor's advice and take something stronger.

Tylenol, aspirin, and ibuprofen are all safe during pregnancy, although aspirin and ibuprofen should be limited as the delivery date approaches. Some prescription medications can also treat headaches. Some drugs even prevent headaches from starting.

People often think of any severe headache as a "migraine," but they are really not the same thing. A migraine usually hurts only on one side of the head. Most people with migraine feel nausea or have photophobia or phonophobia. (Photophobia means that light bothers you or makes the headache worse, and phonophobia means that sound has this bothersome effect.)

Some people with migraines have an "aura"—a visual or other disturbance that tells the person when a migraine is coming. Sufferers of "classic migraine" have these auras while those with "common migraine" do not. Headaches that occur on both sides of the head or are not associated with photophobia, phonophobia, or nausea are technically called "tension headaches," not because tension or stress cause the headache, but rather to distinguish these headaches from migraines. The differences among these types of headaches are not as important as identifying a treatment that works for you.

High estrogen levels may increase migraines. Migraines usually improve during pregnancy when progesterone—rather than estrogen—is the dominant hormone. Birth control pills sometimes help women with menstrual migraine (a headache that comes with every menstrual cycle). Of course, you can't take birth control pills during pregnancy, but there are safe drugs for headaches during pregnancy.

Doctors may encourage their patients to "suffer through" the headache in order to avoid using drug treatments. But women with migraines do not have any higher risk of having a baby with birth defects than do women in the general population—even if the migraine sufferers use prescription medications during pregnancy.

Three kinds of medications may be useful during pregnancy:

Over-the-counter treatments should be the first-line treatment in pregnancy. Acetaminophen (Tylenol) is used most commonly. If this works, great. If not, try either aspirin and ibuprofen. Neither one causes birth defects. Both can result in slight increases in bleeding if taken at delivery and should be avoided when you get within two to four weeks of your due date.

Ibuprofen, taken daily or nearly daily in the third trimester, can reduce the amount of amniotic fluid around the baby. Once-a-week use does not cause this problem.

Consider using these over-the-counter medications in combination with other drugs. Many people with migraine feel nauseated when they have headaches. Combining an over-the-counter analgesic with an antinausea medication can relieve the nausea and improve pain relief. Prochlorperazine (Compazine) and metoclopramide (Reglan) are prescription antinausea medications that are safe during pregnancy.

Combining Tylenol or aspirin with caffeine can also be very effective. Caffeine is safe during pregnancy (see Chapter Six) and helps constrict blood vessels in the head. Dilation of these blood vessels contributes to both tension and migraine headaches, so constricting them helps.

If these over-the-counter treatments don't work, your doctor should help you find a prescription medication that does. Don't suffer just because you are pregnant.

Q: *I've tried the over-the-counter headache remedies and nothing works. What should I do?*

A: Most prescription medications are safe in pregnancy. Of the 3,000 or more drugs licensed by the FDA, fewer than twenty can't be taken during pregnancy.

Codeine, methadone, and morphine present no significant risk to a pregnancy when used to treat headaches. Women who use these drugs to treat their migraine headaches do not have a higher risk of birth defects, stillbirth, or miscarriage. These medications may be habit-forming if taken for long periods of time—but this danger is no greater or less during pregnancy.

Other prescription medications can control migraine, although they do not directly treat pain. Sumatriptan, another drug used specifically to treat migraine, appears to be safe during pregnancy. However, no long-term studies have been done, so it is reserved for headaches that don't respond to treatment with other medications.

Barbiturates (commonly thought of as sleeping pills) can also be used safely during pregnancy to treat occasional migraines. Butalbital, a component of one of the most common combination drugs for migraines (Fiorinal), is a barbiturate. Diazepam (Valium) also has minimal risk during pregnancy and can reduce headaches for some headache sufferers. Both of these drugs, like narcotics, can be addicting so they should be used sparingly.

Suffering through headaches will not improve your pregnancy outcome. Many drugs can and should be used to treat headaches during pregnancy. You should not accept pregnancy as the basis for inadequate treatment.

Q: *Are there any nondrug treatments for headaches?*

A: There are behavioral and nondrug treatments that can help headaches. Doctors at the University of Pittsburgh School of Medicine studied a series of nondrug treatments. These behavioral treatments included relaxation techniques, biofeedback, and physical therapy. The researchers found improved headaches in women who learned these techniques. Unless you live near a major hospital with an integrated headache treatment program, it may be difficult to find someone who can train you in these techniques. Headache support groups in your area or on the Internet, and neurologists who work with pregnant women, may be your best bets for finding treatment resources in your area (see **Resources** for more information.)

Why Do I Look So Good if I Feel So Bad?

5

Morning Sickness and Beyond

"I enjoy convalescence. It is the part that makes the illness worthwhile."—George Bernard Shaw

Being pregnant can be wonderful—but not if you have morning sickness. And if you have the most severe form, called *hyperemesis gravidarum,* it can be devastating. Even mild morning sickness can severely cramp your style, turning an otherwise terrific experience into a trying one. Doctors often advise women to "wait it out," but this advice ignores many simple, safe treatments that can help this difficult condition. The chapter contains practical tips for combating your symptoms. It describes a wide range of treatments, from lifestyle changes to acupuncture to safe medications that can help you battle pregnancy-related nausea. These treatments can help mild nausea go away completely and can even help manage the most severe case—reducing the need for more severe treatments like hospitalization and IVs.

Q: *What causes morning sickness?*

A: Nobody knows, but there are several theories. Psychological explanations rely on evidence that women who are more anxious are more likely to develop morning sickness. Cultural explanations attempt to explain nausea and vomiting as a manifestation of societal factors. Physiological theories depend on relationships between nausea and vomiting and measures of certain hormones, like progesterone or HCG. Genetic theories suppose that inherited characteristics affect one's likelihood of developing morning sickness. Proponents of each of these theories have some facts to back up their case, but nobody has firmly identified the cause.

The history of medicine includes many examples of complex and confusing conditions being labeled as the result of psychological or cultural factors until scientists can identify the true meaningful physical cause. For example, schizophrenia was thought to result from a poor relationship with one's mother but is now recognized as having a biological basis.

It has long been recognized that higher levels of *human chorionic gonadotropin* (HCG), a hormone that is produced by the placenta, are related to an increased risk of severe nausea and vomiting in pregnancy. There has also recently been an intriguing finding in many women with the most severe form of morning sickness (called *hyperemesis gravidarum*). These women are more likely to have the bacteria *Helicobacter pylori* in their stomachs. This is the same bacteria that causes most ulcers. Several doctors have reported treating women with the same antibiotics used to treat ulcers. Some of these women experienced dramatic improvement of their symptoms as a result, but in other cases the antibiotics didn't help at all. Furthermore, many women with morning sickness are not infected with *H. pylori* at all. So, while this "bacterial" theory is being investigated, the bottom line is that as of this writing nobody really knows what causes morning sickness.

Q: *Other than making me feel terrible, is morning sickness really dangerous? I mean, shouldn't I just tough it out?*

A: You shouldn't tough this out any more than you should "tough out" high blood pressure or diabetes. Morning sickness is a real problem. Between fifty and ninety percent of all pregnant women have some degree of morning sickness, and it profoundly impacts many women's lives. Morning sickness can disrupt social activities, interfere with normal relationships, and make it impossible to work. Persistent vomiting leads to dehydration, weakness, and weight loss. Severe nausea can also cause depression, irritability, and difficulty sleeping. Unhelpful friends and coworkers will often share stories about how their nausea was very bad but they just stuck it out until it went away. Half of women do have complete relief of their symptoms by week fourteen to fifteen of pregnancy, but ten percent still have symptoms after twenty-two weeks.

If being sick had no impact on your life, or if the treatments for morning sickness were dangerous, then "toughing it out" would be a good idea. But neither of these things are true. Morning sickness can dramatically interfere with your life. And many treatments have been *proved* safe.

Q: *I can only eat lima beans and tuna fish. Everything else makes me gag. Is this going to hurt my baby somehow?*

A: Aside from being a disgusting diet, there is nothing dangerous about it. One of the theories about morning sickness is that it exerts a protective effect. That is, the "purpose" of nausea in pregnancy is to cause you to avoid foods that could potentially harm your baby. In any event, giving in to your cravings is safe.

The tuna part of your diet is also fine, although as we discuss in Chapter 6 there is some reason to watch your overall fish consumption throughout pregnancy. Certainly, while you're feeling ill, eating tuna even for breakfast, lunch, and dinner offers no danger. But averaged over your entire pregnancy, you probably shouldn't be eating more than a couple of cans a week, as the tiny amount of mercury in the tuna can gradually accumulate in your body.

Women with nausea commonly try to avoid spicy foods, chocolate, coffee, tea, meats, fatty foods, vegetables, and alcohol. On the other hand, many women with morning sickness increase their consumption of fruits, ice cream, carbonated beverages, and meats. There is overlap between what some women avoid and what other women seek out, so there is obviously quite a bit of personal preference involved. For most women, severe nausea peaks between eight and twelve weeks and begins to decline by week fourteen to fifteen, so even severe dietary restrictions for this short period of time should not cause any problems for you or your baby.

Q: *My diet is pretty bad; should I take an extra prenatal vitamin?*

A: It might seem that when you are nauseated and unable to eat a balanced diet that taking prenatal vitamins would be a good idea. It isn't, because they commonly make nausea worse. Instead, try taking only the necessary vitamins and minerals and avoid the multivitamins. Calcium, folic acid, and B6 are the most important ones.

Several studies have shown that twenty-five milligrams of vitamin B6 three times a day *reduces* nausea. (A typical prenatal vitamin contains only about two milligrams of B6.) During the first twelve weeks of pregnancy, you should also take folic acid supplements as they can reduce the risk of spinal cord defects (you probably aren't getting enough folic acid from lima beans and tuna fish). You should also take a calcium supplement—you can take this in Tums®, the antacid, which is largely calcium and may help settle your stomach, or by taking either calcium carbonate or calcium acetate supplements.

Q: *My friend got incredibly sick with her pregnancy. I feel fine and I'm ten weeks pregnant. Does this mean my pregnancy isn't normal?*

A: Absolutely not. Many obstetricians tell their patients who are feeling sick that it's "a good sign," which is true but only to a limited extent. Women with morning sickness early in pregnancy have a slightly lower risk of miscarriage later on. The key word is *slightly;* by no means does the lack of nausea mean you will miscarry. Although between seventy and ninety percent of women have at least some nausea, pregnancies usually turn out fine, even for the lucky minority who don't get sick. Just thank your lucky stars.

Theories Explaining Morning Sickness

1. Psychological: Mental stress produces physical illness.
Evidence: Women who are more anxious are more likely to have morning sickness.

2. Cultural: Women are "trained" to develop morning sickness by what they see and hear.
Evidence: Some cultures have a much lower incidence of morning sickness than we do.

3. Genetic: Some women are born with certain factors that predispose them to developing morning sickness.
Evidence: There is a greater risk of morning sickness in women whose mothers had it.

4. Hormonal: Changes in hormones cause nausea.
Evidence: Sickness peaks when HCG levels are highest.

5. Infectious: Ulcer-causing bacteria multiply during pregnancy causing sickness.
Evidence: Treatment with antiulcer drugs has cured some women.

Note: These are all *theories*. There is no proof that any one theory explains all cases of morning sickness.

Q: *I can hardly get out of bed because of my morning sickness. I don't want to take any medicines because I'm afraid of hurting my baby, but I've lost six pounds already. Are there any herbs that might help me?*

A: One thing is certain: Starving yourself won't help your baby. I understand your desire to do the best thing. But in this case the best thing doesn't mean avoiding medications. The best thing is to stay healthy, and staying healthy when you have morning sickness means taking medications. That's all there is to it. End of story.

Remember that medications (herbal or otherwise) strong enough to make you feel better are also strong enough to hurt you. You need something that helps without posing a risk to you or your baby. Happily there is at least one herb that can help with nausea.

Taking 250 milligrams of ginger four times a day has been scientifically shown to reduce morning sickness. Unfortunately, since the FDA does not regulate ginger (it's considered a food, not a drug), it's very difficult to know how to get the right amount. Ginger has been used as a folk remedy for nausea for a long time, so there are many different ginger preparations available. In studies of ginger for morning sickness, the scientists carefully weighed and measured the ginger to get just the right amount. If you want to get ginger without a supplement, you can try to increase your intake of foods with ginger in them (like gingersnaps, ginger ale, or ginger tea.) If you do this, buy these foods at a health food store because mass-produced gingersnaps and ginger ale generally don't have real ginger in them. Also, you may not get enough ginger to have an effect, so if the ginger ale doesn't do it, consider the supplements.

There is no good research about the safety of other herbs for morning sickness, so I would avoid them. Herbal doesn't mean it's safe: Hemlock and cyanide—two deadly poisons—come from plants.

A terrific resource for anybody interested in herbal products is a book called *Herbal Medicine: Expanded Commission E Monographs.* This book contains fairly comprehensive listings of many different medicinal herbs. For many of the herbs, a section is included describing whether or not the herb has any use in pregnancy, and the herb's safety record. I use this book all the time when women ask about the safety of a particular herb in pregnancy.

Q: *Can changing my diet help my sickness? Some people say to stay away from certain foods, but I eat so few things without getting sick, I'm afraid to give up too much more.*

A: Don't worry. Many women do avoid certain foods when they feel sick, but there is no predetermined list of things to avoid. Preparing certain foods, smelling them, or even thinking about them can make some women nauseated. Coffee sometimes seems to be a common offender on this list, but it's not as if avoiding caffeine "cures" morning sickness. If you've found things that you can enjoy eating without getting sick, then I wouldn't recommend changing anything.

Q: *I hear that acupuncture can help morning sickness but I'm afraid of needles. What should I do?*

A: A variety of studies have proven that *acupressure* is even *better* than acupuncture when it comes to treating nausea in pregnancy. There is an acupressure point called the P6 point located on the wrist (see figure 5). Pressure on this point can relieve even severe morning sickness. One of the first things I recommend to women who are nauseated is to buy Sea Bands, which are sold in marine supply stores (and now many pharmacies). These elastic bracelets have a small plastic button that presses on the P6 acupressure point. These wrist bands have been sold for years to treat seasickness and can be very effective. Studies of acupressure for morning sickness have found that nausea improves in sixty to seventy percent of women who wear these wrist bands.

The band must be properly placed to activate the P6 point. You can find this point by turning your wrist over so that your hand faces the sky, taking the index and middle finger of your other hand and placing them on your wrist so that your middle finger is lying next to the crease of your wrist that is closest to your hand. Then, just below your index finger, in the middle of your wrist, there are two tendons. You can feel these tendons as strong structures running the same direction as the veins in your wrist. Between those tendons, just below your index finger, is the P6 point.

The bands can be worn all day long. It may take several days for the effect to appear but when it does, it is generally dramatic. Many women wear the wrist bands, find that their nausea goes away, and do not believe that it had to do with the bands. They take the wrist bands off and the nausea comes back.

Some studies of acupuncture have shown a benefit in nausea but acupressure bands do just as good a job. Properly done, acupuncture isn't

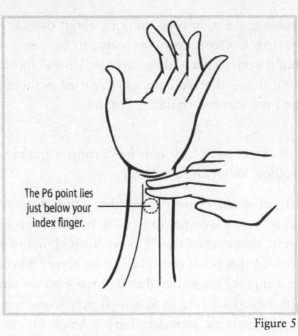

The P6 point lies just below your index finger.

Figure 5

dangerous (even in pregnancy). And since many women do improve with treatment, you may want to consider it. If you do get acupuncture, be sure to tell your acupuncturist that you're pregnant (some acupuncture points can stimulate uterine contractions, although acupuncture does not seem to start labor). As a side note on acupuncture in pregnancy, there was an amazing study several years ago showing that acupuncture on the little toe helped to turn breech (butt down) babies around to a head-first position! (For more details, see Chapter 15.)

Q: *I have tried every remedy my doctor recommended, including small meals, eating before I get out of bed in the morning, avoiding caffeine, taking Tums, and avoiding spicy foods, and I'm still sick. What should I do?*

A: What do you usually do when home remedies don't work? Open the medicine cabinet. There are some completely safe medicines for morning sickness. These drugs have been incredibly well studied and are extremely effective.

The most effective and safest treatment for morning sickness combines two different drugs: vitamin B6, (also called pyridoxine) twenty-five milligrams three times a day, and twenty-five milligrams of the antihistamine doxylamine taken at bedtime. Doxylamine is found in the over-the-counter sleep aid Unisom (twenty-five milligrams is half a tablet). You can take the other half of the tablet in the morning, but it makes some people drowsy. This medication combination can be phenomenally successful at reducing severe nausea and vomiting.

B6 and doxylamine used to be sold as Bendectin, the only drug ever approved in the United States to treat morning sickness. The manufacturer took Bendectin off the market out of fear of lawsuits. The combination is still available in Canada under the name Diclectin. Its safety has been demonstrated over and over again. In a recent study of 17,000 women, the risk of bad outcome was exactly the same for these 17,000 as for 140,000 women in the study who did not take the drug. This is as good a proof of safety as you can get.

The combination of B6 and doxylamine is absolutely the best pharmacological treatment for nausea in pregnancy around. It's safe, it works, and you should try it.

If it fails, and the acupressure and ginger haven't worked either, your choices are a bit more limited. There are other drugs available; most of them require a prescription and if you're sick enough to need them, you need to make sure your doctor has plenty of experience treating women with severe nausea in pregnancy. This can be a difficult condition to treat and being malnourished is certainly not safe for your baby, so make sure your doctor isn't taking it lightly. Drugs that have been safely used in pregnancy include Prochlorperazine (Compazine), promethazine (Phenergan), metoclopramide (Reglan), ondansetron (Zofran), and many others.

Q: A friend in Canada said she took a medicine that really helped her. Why isn't it available in the United States?

A: It's a long and somewhat boring story, so be assured that if you are only interested in curing your sickness and not in a history lesson, you can safely skip this section. Otherwise, read on.

In the late 1950s, Merrell Dow, a large chemical and pharmaceutical company, introduced Bendectin into the market place. This drug combined doxylamine and pyridoxine and was tested and marketed to women who had pregnancy sickness. Several studies supported the effectiveness of this combination in treating this illness. Patient experience bore this out. Hospitalizations for vomiting in pregnancy dropped dramatically after the drug was in widespread use. The drug became increasingly popular and was used by more than 33 million pregnant women by the early 1980s. The drug underwent one formulation change (between 1956 and 1976, it contained an additional ingredient, dicyclomine) but this was removed when it was found to have no effect on nausea.

At around the same time that Bendectin was introduced, another drug called Thalidomide was introduced in West Germany. This too was designed to combat morning sickness. Use of Thalidomide rapidly spread to other countries in Europe, Asia, Australia, and North America. Within a few years, an Australian gynecologist began to suspect that Thalidomide caused certain types of limb deformities. Doctors in Australia and West Germany eventually became convinced that Thalidomide was to blame for a rash of cases of phocomelia. This literally means "seal limb." Babies born with phocomelia have their hands directly attached to the shoulder or the foot directly to the hip without a leg or arm between. Thalidomide was withdrawn from the markets in West Germany and the United Kingdom in 1961, and from Canadian markets in early 1962. It was never sold in the United States.

In the late 1960s and early 1970s, victims of the Thalidomide tragedy and their families brought legal action against the companies that manufactured and distributed the drugs. They often received cash payments and annual payments that continued throughout their lives because of their disability.

Merrell Dow, concerned that similar lawsuits would be financially devastating, decided in 1983 to withdraw Bendectin from the U.S. market. Bendectin was never associated with any type of abnormality: not major limb deformities like Thalidomide, not miscarriages, not even minor and reversible problems at birth. Nor did Dow ever have to pay out a single claim based on the use of Bendectin. Rather, they decided that rather than face accusers in court, they would withdraw the drug. Remember that as many as one in ten pregnant women took this drug combination at some point in their pregnancies during the years it was available. Of course, some of these women would have had babies with deformities (since about one in 300 babies has some type of birth defect). Dow did not want to face the possibility of trying to defend itself in court when a woman stood opposite them with a deformed baby.

After Bendectin was withdrawn from the market, the hospitalization rate for women with severe nausea of pregnancy skyrocketed. Subsequent studies of the deformity rate in babies, both before and after Bendectin was on the market, demonstrate fairly conclusively that this drug does not cause birth defects. As a result, it has been called the most famous non-teratogen ever.

Bendectin is still available in Canada under the trade name Diclectin. A comprehensive review by the Canadian Health Service in 1989 determined that there was "no measurable risk" of Diclectin on pregnancy and it continues to be available there. There have been some recent rumblings that the drug would be reintroduced into the American market but this has not yet occurred.

Q: *My doctor says I need to go into the hospital because of my morning sickness but I have three other kids at home. How can I make sure I get home quickly?*

A: You don't have morning sickness, you have *hyperemesis gravidarum* (see **When Is It More Than Morning Sickness?** below). This is a severe illness that may be the most severe form of morning sickness but also may represent an entirely different problem. Women with hyperemesis gravidarum can't keep liquids down and have disturbances of their body chemistry. Their body weight drops by more than five percent, and they will have abnormalities detectable on blood testing. Unlike typical morning sickness, hyperemesis lasts throughout an entire pregnancy (it is sometimes not even diagnosed until after most women have stopped having typical morning sickness—about fourteen or fifteen weeks of pregnancy).

Hyperemesis gravidarum is devastating to the women who have it, and to their families. Many women get so sick that they choose to have abortions rather than continue their pregnancy. Hyperemesis gravidarum requires hospitalization and treatment with IV nutritional therapy as well

When Is It More Than Morning Sickness?

Doctors use the term *hyperemesis gravidarum* to describe very severe pregnancy sickness.

- *Hyper* means too much
- *Emesis* means vomiting
- *Gravid* means pregnant

Characteristics of hyperemesis gravidarum:

- Changes in levels of blood electrolytes—these chemicals (sodium and potassium among others) can become unbalanced by repeated vomiting—this can only be seen with a blood test.
- Presence of *ketones* in the blood. The body produces ketones when it doesn't have enough food. They are evidence of starvation and can only be seen with a blood test.
- Weight loss and/or need for intravenous fluids. Most women with hyperemesis must be hospitalized to get fluids.

as treatment with a variety of prescription medications. There is no completely satisfactory cure, but it is clearly worth treating with the strongest medications available. Many medications have been used for years in pregnancy and have been determined to be safe enough to treat this very difficult condition. Many would not be recommended as first-line treatments for morning sickness simply because not enough data exist about their safety in pregnancy. But when somebody is hospitalized, throwing up constantly, and losing weight, then the risk/benefit ratio changes. In this case, medications for which there is less evidence of safety should be used.

This is not a condition that should be treated by somebody who sees only one case a year. Make sure that your doctor has plenty of experience treating hyperemesis and if he or she doesn't, seek out expert advice. There are organizations devoted to helping doctors and patients deal with hyperemesis (see **Resources** section). You can find others on the Internet or by asking in your doctor's office.

Coping With Morning Sickness

Diet Changes

- Eat small, frequent meals
- Eat something before getting out of bed
- Avoid spicy foods if they bother you
- Avoid caffeine if it makes your nausea worse

Safe Medications/Herbs

- Ginger 250 milligrams four times a day
- Vitamin B6 (pyridoxine) 25 milligrams three times a day
- Doxylamine (found in Unisom) 25 milligrams at night

Safe Alternatives

- Acupuncture by a licensed provider
- Acupressure
- Acupressure wrist bands (Sea Bands®)

Q: *I'm still sick and I'm in my fifth month. Doesn't it ever go away?*

A: It does go away, but for some women, it takes longer than for others. About one in seven women with pregnancy sickness has symptoms that last beyond twenty weeks. By about twenty-four weeks of pregnancy, the number of women still suffering drops to one in ten.

For some women, nausea of pregnancy simply can't be controlled with any of the known treatments. In the United States, however, the most common reason for persistent nausea is inadequate treatment. Make sure your doctor has considered all the various treatments outlined above. Don't ignore any potential solutions to your problem—even if you don't believe that things like herbs or acupuncture could help, they might be worth a try. Don't let your continued illness be a reflection of an unwillingness on the part of you or your doctor to try something new. If all these treatments fail, then you may just have to wait it out.

6 Life Without Starbucks?

Food and Drink in Pregnancy

"I never drink coffee at lunch. I find it keeps me awake for the afternoon."—Ronald Reagan

Eating a healthy diet may sound simple, but most of us don't eat nearly as well as we should. Americans rely too much on fast foods and snack foods. Pregnant women often wonder what effect their less-than-perfect diets have on pregnancy. This chapter helps separate diet facts from fiction. Does the typical American diet increase your risks of problems with pregnancy? For example, most American women start their day with a cup of coffee. In the past few years, news reports have scared many pregnant women away from this habit. This chapter reviews the evidence and concludes that coffee is much safer than many women think. Other food taboos are similarly unfounded; that pregnant women should avoid Caesar salads and sushi are two of the more common food myths. Among other topics, this chapter addresses the safety and effects on pregnancy of consuming artificial sweeteners, dyes, preservatives, and milk from cows given hormones.

Q: *I haven't had a cup of coffee since I got pregnant but I still drink tea. Is this safe?*

A: Yes, it is. Caffeine in large amounts may increase the risk of early miscarriage. But, according to the Organization of Teratology Information Services (a scientific organization that studies birth defects, see

Resources), even large amounts of caffeine do not increase the risk of birth defects. (For more information, visit www.otispregnancy.org.) Caffeine intake is measured in milligrams—one cup of coffee has between seventy-five and 150 milligrams of caffeine, while espresso has about 150 milligrams per serving (as does coffee from Starbucks). Tea has about thirty milligrams per cup and caffeinated cola drinks have about fifty milligrams per cup. Caffeine consumption of 300 milligrams a day or less has never been linked to *any* pregnancy-related problems.

Some studies show that women who consume more than 300 milligrams of caffeine a day on average (that means *more* than four typical cups of coffee) had about a twenty percent higher rate of spontaneous miscarriage before twelve weeks. Another study showed heavy coffee drinkers had slightly smaller babies.

Caffeine does not cause preterm labor. Other studies show no impact of caffeine until levels reach 800 milligrams a day (about two "venti" coffees at Starbucks).

I recommend keeping your caffeine intake to below 300 milligrams a day. Notice that I don't say stop drinking coffee. There is no reason,

Caffeine Content of Common Foods*

Try to stay below 300 milligrams a day *on average* (600 milligrams one day followed by zero milligrams the next is fine).

Coffee:	sixty-five to 150 milligrams per eight ounce cup
Tea:	twenty to thirty-five milligrams per eight ounce cup
Coca Cola:	forty-five milligrams per 250 milliliter can
Coffee ice cream:	forty to sixty milligrams per cup
Chocolate:	ten to fifteen milligrams per bar
Hot chocolate	five to ten milligrams per cup
Excedrin	130 milligrams in two tablets
Guarana	forty milligrams per capsule

*Caffeine content varies significantly from one particular brand to another; therefore, these numbers are only approximations.

based on the science, to stop drinking caffeinated drinks entirely. Telling women to stop drinking coffee completely is no different than saying "since too much vitamin A can make you sick, you should avoid vitamin A entirely." And remember, even the highest levels of caffeine consumption only increase the risk of having a miscarriage by a small amount. I don't think it's crazy to accept that small risk if you feel the need for five or six cups of coffee a day.

I can hardly imagine being able to leave my house without a cup of coffee. It's a feeling I wouldn't wish on anybody, pregnant or not.

Q: *Can I eat sushi during pregnancy?*

A: You sure can. I find this very common misconception all over the Internet and hear it passed from woman to woman. I've heard women say, "Oh my God, I'm dying for some sushi, but I know I can't have any because I'm pregnant." A pregnant friend once told me, "Well, we can go out for sushi but I have to stick to the cooked stuff and the vegetarian rolls."

There is nothing in sushi that is dangerous to your baby. Sure, you can get sick from eating sushi. Cooking foods kills parasites and bacteria that can cause illness. If you're going to eat raw foods, you're going to face an increased risk of infection. This is why our ancestors learned that fire was a good thing. But those infection risks are for *you*, the mom, not the baby.

What's the worst thing that's going to happen from eating sushi? You're going to get a parasite. Now, that's no fun, but it surely isn't dangerous for your baby. Unless, of course, you fail to treat the parasite because you're so worried that the treatment will hurt your baby (which it won't) and you become malnourished.

There have also been cases of hepatitis A from uncooked fish. But again, these are the same risks that you faced eating sushi before you got pregnant. If they didn't bother you then, why do they bother you now? Neither hepatitis A nor parasites can be passed from mother to fetus. (You can even be vaccinated against hepatitis A during pregnancy.)

"Well," women say, "I just don't want to take any extra risks while

I'm pregnant." That's fine. You're certainly entitled to change your dietary habits when you're pregnant. But don't do it because you think you're avoiding some risk to your baby. If it makes you feel better to not go outside during the daytime when you're pregnant because you're afraid that solar radiation is going to cause damage to your fetus and you just want to "play it safe," feel free. Just don't kid yourself that you're doing it based on any kind of rational or scientific evidence.

Just so you don't think this is my crazy rant, the next time somebody tells you to avoid sushi because you're pregnant, refer them to the Centers for Disease Control (CDC) in Atlanta, or to the Food and Drug Administration (FDA) (see **Resources** for the CDC and FDA websites). These organizations identify food- and infection-related risks for pregnant women. Neither one considers sushi worth warning women about. If you want to avoid something, avoid lox. There have been a few cases of listeria infection in smoked salmon and listeria actually can harm your baby (see below).

Q: *Somebody told me that I shouldn't eat feta cheese or yogurt during pregnancy because of the bacteria. Is that true?*

A: It's true for certain kinds of feta cheese but not for yogurt. While both of these foods may contain bacteria, there is an important distinction between the kind of bacteria found in them.

Yogurt generally contains *Lactobacillus acidophilus* bacteria. This bacteria commonly lives in the intestinal tract and can actually be good for you. There is no link of any kind between eating yogurt and problems with pregnancy. In fact, yogurt is high in calcium and (if unflavored) relatively low in simple sugars.

Feta cheese made with unpasteurized milk, on the other hand, may be contaminated with a bacteria known as *Listeria monocytogenes*. If the feta carries a label saying that it's pasteurized, it won't have any listeria in it. Most people who get listeria develop headaches, nausea, diarrhea, and fever. (People with compromised immune systems, like those with HIV, can have even more serious consequences, including death.) Listeria can harm pregnant women because it is one of the few infections that can cross through the placenta and into the fetus. (Others include chicken pox, toxoplasmosis, and parvovirus.) Fetal listeria infection can cause miscarriage, preterm delivery, and fetal death.

Before you get too worried, you should know that listeria infections are extremely rare. According to the Centers for Disease Control, fewer than twenty pregnant women in the entire country get listeria infection each year.

Nonetheless, most pregnant women want to avoid even the *smallest* risk and you can do this by taking the CDC's simple precautions:

- Do not eat hot dogs and luncheon meats unless they are steaming hot.

- Do not eat soft cheeses like feta, brie, and camembert, unless they are labeled as being made with pasteurized milk.

- Do not eat refrigerated patés or meat spreads (canned or prepackaged spreads are safe).

- Do not eat refrigerated smoked seafood such as lox, smoked salmon, smoked trout, or smoked white fish. (Canned smoked seafood is safe.)

- Do not drink raw or unpasteurized milk.

If you develop diarrhea, headache, nausea and vomiting during pregnancy, you should see your doctor, although it is extraordinarily unlikely that you have listeria.

Q: *I usually eat steaks rare. Is that safe now that I'm pregnant?*

A: Pregnant women face no more risk from a rare steak than do nonpregnant women. Cooking food, particularly to high temperatures, does kill bacteria. And the more bacteria in food, the higher the risk of infection. So very rare steak carries a slightly higher risk of infection than does well-done steak. But this risk is no higher because you're pregnant. The most common infection seen from rare steak is with the bacteria *Escherichia coli*. *E. coli* does not cross the placenta, so even if you get infected, your baby will not.

If you are concerned about *E. coli* infection, then I would recommend not eating rare steak *ever*. There is no reason to make a different recommendation for pregnant women than for nonpregnant ones.

Q: *I heard that I shouldn't eat Caesar salad while I'm pregnant. Is it true?*

A: Caesar salad traditionally contains raw egg in the dressing; egg can harbor salmonella and salmonella can make you sick. This is another case where the sickness you would get would be no different whether you were pregnant or not. So the advice to avoid Caesar salad, if it's good advice (and I'm not saying it is), should apply to *everyone*.

Salmonella infection does not cross the placenta and therefore presents no risk to your fetus. Generally, salmonella is a very mild infection causing no more than diarrhea (although it can be worse). Furthermore, the risk of salmonella in uncooked eggs has dropped dramatically over the years. Only one in 20,000 eggs has any salmonella bacteria in it at all. Couple this with the fact that most exposures to salmonella don't result in illness, and you could eat Caesar salad from morning to night every day of your pregnancy and probably not get sick.

Q: *I'm going to Europe. Is there anything I should worry about as far as food goes?*

A: There is no particular risk of any single European food greater than that of its American equivalent. Safety standards in Europe are quite high. In many instances, food standards in the European Union are higher than those in the United States. For example, the European Union has very strict rules on genetically modified food, whereas the United States has no such rules. There have been reports of outbreaks of listeria in Europe, particularly in France, but these all appeared to be related to foods on the CDC's list that pregnant women should avoid. (See **Foods To Avoid During Pregnancy.**)

Foods to Avoid During Pregnancy

- More than three cups of coffee a day
- Tile fish, swordfish, king mackerel, and shark
- Cold hot dogs and luncheon meats
- Soft cheeses like brie, feta, and camembert (if made with unpasteurized milk)
- Refrigerated patés or meat spreads
- Unpasteurized milk
- Refrigerated smoked seafood

If you avoid foods on this list, you should be quite safe. (See **Resources** for more sources of food safety information.)

Q: *My girlfriend told me that she only buys food in the organic section of the grocery store. Is this important to be sure I have a healthy baby?*

A: No, you shouldn't do it for your baby's health, but you may want to do it for your own health. Thanks to a ten-year-old federal law that was only recently fully implemented, foods bearing the label "100 percent organic" cannot contain any pesticides, petroleum-based fertilizers, or sewage sludge fertilizers. Animals that are labeled "100 percent organic" must be given organic feed and access to the outdoors. They cannot be given antibiotics or growth hormones to improve the speed at which they develop. Some products may also be labeled "organic" rather than "100 percent organic" and these must contain at least ninety-five percent organically produced ingredients.

Foods That Are Safe During Pregnancy

- Sushi
- Foods containing dyes or preservatives
- Yogurt with live yogurt cultures
- Tuna (up to three 4-ounce servings a week)
- Sodas or other products with artificial sweeteners
- Caesar salad

Organic foods have fewer pesticides and pesticide byproducts in them. While there is no conclusive information linking pesticide byproducts to problems with human health, many studies have suggested such a link.

Organic foods are also produced with fewer antibiotics.

Overuse of antibiotics in livestock and poultry has been an alarming problem; more antibiotics are given to cows in this country than to people, and antibiotics are included in livestock feed whether or not the animals are sick, and these antibiotics vastly increase the risk of antibiotic resistance. Antibiotic resistance (in both livestock and people) has risen sharply over the past several decades and is beginning to present a significant health risk. People infected with resistant bacteria may become desperately ill and can't be treated with the usual antibiotics. Reducing this problem is probably a good enough reason to choose organic products if possible.

That said, there is no reason to believe that organic products are going to improve the likelihood of good pregnancy outcome. It's a choice that you should make based on factors other than pregnancy.

If you choose *not* to buy organic, rest assured that pesticides have never been shown to be harmful to pregnancy. Even studies examining women at the highest risk from pesticides, for example women who work in agricultural occupations, do not conclusively show any problems. If the cost of organics bothers you, you can remove most pesticide residue by washing fruits and vegetables with a mild soap solution. Just put a few drops of soap in a basin of water and thoroughly wash the skin before you cook or eat vegetables.

Q: *Is milk from cows treated with hormones safe to drink while pregnant?*

A: Many cows are now treated with recombinant bovine growth hormone (sometimes called *bovine somatotropin* or BST) in order to increase milk output and profits for dairy farmers. There is absolutely no benefit to the milk drinker from this treatment, and increasing the use of hormones in our food seems like a terrible idea to me, so I don't buy milk from cows treated with BST.

That said, there is no evidence that BST treatment is risky to the milk drinker—pregnant or not. No BST gets into the milk, so BST itself isn't a problem. There are subtle differences between milk from cows treated with this drug and milk from untreated cows, but it seems pretty unlikely that these differences could harm a pregnancy. Over the long run, it's conceivable that these changes could have some impact on a milk drinker, but it's doubtful that they would affect a fetus. The best argument for avoiding milk from BST-treated cows is that the only problem it solves is low profits for milk producers.

Q: *My doctor told me to drink lots of water. Why is that so important? Does it have to be bottled water?*

A: Don't get me started. The issue of how much water pregnant women (or anybody) should drink is a pet peeve of mine. When I was in medical school, I noticed that many people carried around bottles of water and drank from them throughout the day. When I asked why, they said it helped with weight loss. Later in my career, I asked several professors why drinking so much water was so important. Most had no idea. Some said simply that good health "required" continually drinking large amounts of water. They couldn't point to any research to support this statement, but insisted it was true.

When I was training to practice obstetrics, I saw doctors giving this same advice to pregnant patients. One of my professors wrote on every prenatal chart how much water the patient was drinking. She encouraged them to increase it until they were drinking eight glasses a day. I wanted to look into the real science behind this advice, but I was too busy catching up on sleep and trying not to forget what my family looked like.

I've finally waited long enough for somebody to do the work for me. In 2002, a professor at Dartmouth Medical School published a comprehensive study of the "eight glasses a day" advice. Professor Heinz Valtin successfully traced back the origins of the statement that people "should drink eight glasses, eight ounces each" of water every day to a 1945 pamphlet from the Food and Nutrition Board of the National Research Council. Without citing any supporting research, the pamphlet said, "a suitable allowance of water for adults is 2.5 liters daily." Furthermore, the very next sentence says "most of this quantity is contained in prepared foods."

Not only is there no research to support the idea that everyone needs sixty-four ounces of water a day, but the water a person *does* need can come largely from foods (apples, lettuce, strawberries, cucumbers, and melons are predominantly water).

Dr. Valtin carefully refutes each and every argument made for why people need to drink an arbitrary amount of water each day. He draws extensively on both his own research and the research of others to show how well the body regulates its own fluid balance. The idea that "by the time you're thirsty, it's too late" also seems to be false. Careful studies show that most people get thirsty well before changes in their body chemistry indicate "dehydration."

Pregnant women are really no different. There is no reason to enforce an arbitrary standard of water drinking on a normal, healthy, pregnant woman. Pregnant women need more fluids, but they are more thirsty as well. Thirst is what leads to an increased fluid intake—conscious goals (e.g., "eight glasses a day") are unnecessary. If you're not thirsty, you've probably had enough to drink.

The body is a magical and complex machine. It is self-regulating and most of the time, following your body's urges is all you need to do. Drinking water falls into this category. Next time your doctor (or anyone else) tells you to "drink more water," bet them twenty dollars that they can't find any research to back it up. You'll win every time.

Q: *I heard that I shouldn't eat peanuts while I'm pregnant. What could the reason for that possibly be?*

A: Strangely enough, women who eat peanuts during pregnancy are more likely to have children with peanut allergies. In one study, women who ate peanuts or products containing peanuts more than once a week had three times the odds of having a child with peanut allergy. Peanut allergies are becoming more and more common. One possible explanation is that foods containing small amounts of peanuts are becoming more popular. Many processed or prepared foods contain small amounts of peanuts and women eat more of these foods during pregnancy than ever before.

Reducing your intake of peanuts and peanut-containing products during pregnancy might not be a bad idea. On the other hand, the studies that link these two things are far from conclusive. Furthermore, peanuts are a healthful source of protein, so if it's a choice between cheeseburgers and peanuts, the peanuts may be the way to go. The evidence of peanut allergy resulting from maternal consumption is not yet good enough to make a blanket recommendation.

Q: *I've heard that mercury in fish can be dangerous, and that the FDA says pregnant women shouldn't eat fish. Do I have to give up my tuna sandwiches?*

A: No. The most dangerous thing about your tuna sandwich might be the mayonnaise because it can spoil if left unrefrigerated.

The U.S. Center for Food Safety has recommended that pregnant women not eat certain types of fish because of mercury contamination, but tuna is not on this list.

Mercury, although found naturally in the environment, can be dangerous. Mercury levels are higher in areas where there is industrial pollution. Small organisms in the ocean absorb mercury from seawater. Fish take in mercury by eating these organisms. Because the basic food of many larger fish is small fish, mercury levels can increase as you move up the food chain. Long-lived fish tend to have the highest mercury levels. Salmon, oysters, and shrimp have almost undetectable levels of mercury, whereas tuna, grouper, and lobster have about one-half to one-third as much mercury as the fish on the FDA's prohibited list.

The FDA lists four kinds of fish that should be taken off of a pregnant woman's diet completely: tile fish, swordfish, king mackerel, and shark. These fish eat other fish and have the highest mercury levels.

Tuna has relatively low levels of mercury, but because it is so popular the FDA provides guidelines for tuna as well. The FDA currently suggests that pregnant women not eat more than twelve ounces of any canned fish a week on a regular basis. Notice the phrase "on a regular basis"? Mercury accumulates slowly and blood levels depend on the quantity of mercury taken in over many months. The FDA specifically notes that the average shouldn't be more than twelve ounces per week. Not that going over the twelve-ounce limit in one week is dangerous. Rather that over the course of an entire pregnancy, you should consume less than thirty pounds of fish. That's right, thirty pounds. If you're eating this much fish, I think you need to worry more about having the urge to swim up river to spawn than you do about getting too much mercury.

Q: *My mother says that eating liver in pregnancy will help me stay strong. I think this is a trick to get me to eat something she could never force on me as a kid. What do you say?*

A: You can safely skip the liver and I promise the outcome of your pregnancy will be unaffected.

Liver, particularly pork liver, is very high in *heme* iron, the best-absorbed type of iron, and pregnant women do need iron. The FDA recommends that pregnant women get an average of thirty milligrams of elemental iron a day during pregnancy (twice the usual requirement of fifteen milligrams a day). One serving of pork liver provides fifteen milligrams of elemental iron, but liver also has high levels of vitamin A, which may not be such a good thing during pregnancy.

High doses of vitamin A during the first few weeks of pregnancy can cause birth defects. Vitamin A (also known as retinol) is closely related to Retin-A (tretinoin), one of the few medications known to cause birth defects (see Chapter 2). As a result, I don't recommend eating liver on a daily basis in the first few weeks of pregnancy. There are other ways of getting enough dietary iron and a list of iron content of both animal and nonanimal sources is included below.

Q: *I usually drink diet sodas, but now I'm worried about the effect of saccharine on the baby. Are artificial sweeteners safe during pregnancy?*

A: Yes, they are. Even in unusual cases where women have taken massive doses of artificial sweeteners (usually in misguided suicide attempts) there have been no reported cases of toxicity to a fetus. Of the artificial sweeteners, my patients have been most concerned about nonnutritive sweeteners (like saccharine or aspartame), so I'll focus on these, although *none* of the artificial sweeteners are dangerous during pregnancy.

Saccharine is the most controversial, mostly because some studies performed more than thirty years ago found an increase in bladder cancer in rats fed high doses of saccharine. These results were never seen in humans. This sweetener does not raise the risk of bladder cancer. Diabetics have used saccharine for many years without evidence of adverse effects.

Saccharine does cross the placenta and has been measured in the fetus. This should not be alarming—many chemicals cross the placenta without causing damage. There is no reason to think that saccharine (in any amount) is dangerous to your unborn child.

Aspartame is also safe during pregnancy. Scientists have studied this sweetener in detail because it is dangerous to people with *phenylketonuria* (PKU). PKU is extremely rare and is usually diagnosed at birth. People with it are very sensitive to phenylalanine, one of the compo-

Good General Advice for Healthier Eating

- Eat a variety of foods from the five food groups (breads and cereals, fruits and vegetables, meat, fish and other sources of protein, milk and dairy products, and foods with fat or sugar).
- Get 400 milligrams a day of folic acid from your diet, or take a supplement. Good dietary sources of folate include Brussels sprouts (100 micrograms per serving), spinach (80 micrograms per serving), green beans (50 micrograms), fortified breads or grains (50 to 100 micrograms per serving).
- Avoid foods that might be infected with listeria, including soft cheeses (brie and camembert) or blue vein cheeses (Stilton, gorgonzola and Roquefort), paté unless it's canned, and processed luncheon meats or hot dogs unless they are steaming hot.
- Limit your intake of liver to no more than once a day during the first few weeks of pregnancy because of the high vitamin A content.
- Consider avoiding peanuts. Eating them during pregnancy may increase your child's risk of peanut allergies.
- Don't smoke.
- Reduce your coffee drinking to four or fewer cups a day.
- Limit alcohol to no more than two drinks in any given day.

nents of aspartame. If you have PKU, you shouldn't use aspartame, pregnant or not. No one with PKU gets to be an adult without knowing they have the disease. If you don't have PKU, there is no reason to avoid aspartame during pregnancy.

Q: *Are food dyes and preservatives dangerous to my baby's health?*

A: There are no known food dyes or preservatives approved by the FDA that pregnant women need to avoid. In many cases, preserved foods are safer than non-preserved ones are because preservatives reduce the risk of spoilage. Food dyes are cosmetic and don't change the safety of food products one way or another. If you wish to avoid them, you can do so by carefully reading labels.

7 In Sickness and In Health

Infections and Other Illnesses

Everyone hates getting sick. But during pregnancy even the most minor illness raises a new concern: Will this hurt my baby? Infections—from colds and flu to chickenpox—are the most common illnesses women get while pregnant.

Pregnant women get sick in other ways, too. Diabetes, high blood pressure, and depression can begin or worsen during pregnancy. This chapter explains what you need to know to handle the most common, and some less common, illnesses during pregnancy. It explains which illnesses should be treated and how—paying particular attention to which medications are safe to take and which should be avoided. Surprisingly, the best treatments during pregnancy are usually the same ones that work outside of pregnancy—and they're generally completely safe.

Q: I'm afraid of being exposed to colds during pregnancy. What can I do to keep myself safe?

A: Frequent hand washing is the best strategy for avoiding colds. Washing your hands kills virus particles and is the only thing proven to reduce colds. Don't use antibacterial soap—colds come from viruses (not bacteria) and antibacterial soaps probably contribute to the growing problem of antibiotic resistance (that is, these soaps actually make it *harder* to get rid of infections in the long run).

Limiting contact with sick people can reduce your risk of colds. But people with colds can transmit their infection before they develop symptoms, so it's difficult to know whom to avoid. Cold viruses change constantly; that's why having one cold doesn't keep you from getting another one. Cold viruses move through the air; when someone with a cold coughs or sneezes, small mucous droplets are emitted. Each droplet contains up to a million virus particles. If only four or five reach the inside of your nose, mouth, or eyes, you can catch the cold.

Cold viruses can also pass from the inside of someone's nose onto their hands. From there, the virus can move to your hands, and then from your hands to your nose. Once the virus gets to the inside of your nose, you're sick. You won't get a cold from things like doorknobs, money, or public restrooms because cold viruses can't survive outside the body for very long.

According to the National Institute of Allergy and Infectious Diseases, adults get about four colds a year and children get six to twelve. Colds are no more dangerous to you now than before you got pregnant. Cold viruses cannot be passed to your fetus, do not cause birth defects, and do not cause any other pregnancy complications. On the other hand, having a cold when you're pregnant is just a *bit* more miserable than having it when you're not, since your body is already going through so many changes, so you should take some simple precautions like washing your hands frequently and avoiding sick people when possible.

If you do get a cold, you can treat your symptoms the same way you would when you were not pregnant. Tylenol, nasal decongestants, echinacea, zinc, and vitamin C are all safe during pregnancy. Taken in the recommended doses, all the common, over-the-counter cough and cold medications are safe during pregnancy. (More details in Chapter 4.) These treatments probably won't shorten your cold much (if at all) but they may help you feel better. Cold symptoms usually last one to two weeks—so hang in there.

Nondrug cold treatments may also help. Use a saline nasal spray (available in the drug store) to keep your nasal passages clear. Hot soup (chicken or otherwise) makes many people feel better when they have colds. Hot showers can also help open your sinuses if they're blocked.

Q: *Should I get a flu shot during pregnancy? The information sheet the pharmacist gave me says not to, but my doctor recommended it.*

A: Your doctor is right: You should most definitely get a flu shot. People sometimes think "flu" means vomiting and stomach illness, but these are not common symptoms. Flu (properly called influenza) is a viral infection of the upper respiratory tract, and is a disabling illness. People who get the flu have high fevers, headaches, chills, and coughs, and often can't get out of bed for days.

Influenza is very contagious and is transmitted by the coughs and sneezes of the infected person. Most people have flu infections for several days before they develop symptoms, so simply avoiding people who are sick is not a sufficient way to reduce your risk of exposure. During pregnancy, influenza can be an even worse illness than when not pregnant. Women who develop flu during pregnancy are more likely to end up in the hospital with heart or lung problems than nonpregnant women who get it. It's possible, although not proven, that influenza

Safe and Unsafe Vaccines During Pregnancy

Vaccine	Recommendation
Influenza	Recommended (some doctors prefer not to give before three months, but can safely be given at any time in pregnancy).
Rubella	Not recommended during pregnancy.
Mumps	Not recommended during pregnancy.
Chicken pox (varicella)	Not recommended during pregnancy.
Measles	Not recommended during pregnancy.
Hepatitis A	Consider if traveling to high-risk area during pregnancy (see www.cdc.gov for map of these areas).
Hepatitis B	Recommended for most adults. Pregnancy and breastfeeding are *not* reasons to avoid this vaccine.

during pregnancy can increase the risk of miscarriage. Having the flu while you're pregnant won't increase the risk of birth defects.

Flu vaccine is very safe, even during pregnancy and breast feeding. Vaccines to avoid during pregnancy are those that contain live viruses. The influenza vaccine is made of "killed" viruses. It is not infectious and cannot cause the flu—in you or in your baby.

Current recommendations for flu vaccine are that all women who will be in the second or third trimesters during the flu season should receive the vaccine. Flu vaccines usually contain virus particles from three different types of influenza, and the types are updated every year to provide protection against the most common strains. Flu shots must be repeated every year so if you had one last year, it won't help you now.

The flu vaccine has very few side effects, the most common being soreness at the site of injection. Some people report low-grade fever, headache, or a general feeling of discomfort or uneasiness for several days after the flu vaccine but in careful studies, these feelings are no more common than among people who are injected with a placebo.

The vaccine should not be given to anyone who is allergic to eggs because there are egg proteins in it. Flu season usually begins in December and flu vaccines are available beginning in late September or early October. Protection begins almost immediately after receiving the injection, so even if it is well after the beginning of flu season, you should consider the vaccine.

Q: *I'm an elementary school teacher and I've never had chicken pox. What should I do if there's an outbreak in my classroom while I'm pregnant?*

A: The first thing to do is check whether or not you've actually had chicken pox. Everybody who remembers having had chicken pox as a child has most definitely had it. But many people who don't remember having had it (or whose parents don't remember them having it) actually did—and are therefore immune.

Varicella zoster virus (VZV), which causes chicken pox, can sometimes cause a mild infection that does not give you any "pox." People who have had this mild type of infection may not remember having had the illness, but are still immune. If you're not sure, ask your doctor for a blood test to check.

Varicella zoster virus is one of the few viruses that can cross the placenta and cause damage to the fetus. About two out of every 100 women who get chicken pox during pregnancy will have a baby with congenital varicella syndrome. This syndrome includes abnormalities of the limbs, eyes, skin, and brain. Getting chicken pox while pregnant increases the risk of preterm delivery as well.

If you don't know your history and are exposed to chicken pox for the first time during pregnancy, you should get tested as soon as you can. If you are not immune, talk to your doctor about getting *varicella zoster immune globulin* (VZIG). VZIG blocks the chicken pox virus from multiplying in your body. If you take it within four days of exposure, it may prevent you from catching chicken pox. Even if it does not prevent *you* from getting infected, it will reduce your baby's risk. VCIG is very safe. If more than four days have passed since your exposure, you should still consider taking it: The risks are low and the potential benefit is high.

Chicken pox vaccine has been a standard part of childhood immunizations since the mid-1990s. Outbreaks of chicken pox among school-age children are becoming less and less common. This should mean that fewer and fewer pregnant women are exposed to the varicella virus during their pregnancy. Nonetheless, if you are considering getting pregnant and are not sure whether you are immune to chicken pox or not, you should see your doctor and ask to be tested. If you're not immune, you can be given the varicella vaccine *before* you get pregnant.

You should *not* get vaccinated against chicken pox while you are pregnant. The vaccine contains a weakened but still living strain of varicella virus. Because the virus is still alive, it could cross the placenta and infect your baby. Varicella vaccine is sometimes given by mistake to pregnant women who are supposed to be receiving VZIG instead. If your doctor recommends VZIG, ask the person giving the shot to double check that they are giving the proper medication.

Q: *Does it matter how far along I am if I'm exposed to chicken pox?*

A: Yes. Your baby is at the highest risk from chicken pox if you are in your second trimester. At this point, your baby has a one in fifty chance of getting infected. The risk is only one in 500 if you're infected during the first trimester.

If you do develop signs of chicken pox, your doctor should consider giving you acyclovir, a drug that fights varicella infection. Acyclovir appears safe in pregnancy, and lowers the risk of varicella pneumonia. This deadly complication of chicken pox affects pregnant women much more often than other people.

If you get chicken pox more than a week before you deliver, your newborn will probably be protected by the antibodies your body makes, which are passed to the baby. But if you get chicken pox in the few days before you deliver, you baby has a high risk of infection. At this point, the baby won't develop birth defects (because it's fully developed) but babies can become seriously ill from varicella infection. Such infections rarely occur, but your baby will likely need treatment with acyclovir or with other similar drugs.

Q: *I know that I never had chicken pox as a child (I was tested) and my friend has developed shingles. Isn't this the same as chicken pox and can I catch it from her?*

A: It's possible you could, but it's not very likely. The virus that causes chicken pox causes shingles as well. Shingles is a "reactivation infection." It comes from a varicella virus that has been dormant or "sleeping" in someone's body. Shingles is much less infectious than chicken pox. You are not likely to catch it unless you have very close contact with the shingles rash (like rubbing or touching the rash). If you have done this, consider getting *varicella immune globulin* (VZIG). VZIG is safe in pregnancy and could lower your risk of infection.

Women who develop chicken pox despite treatment with VZIG should be treated with acyclovir to reduce their symptoms. Symptoms in pregnant women include not only the pox but potentially pneumonia

Chicken Pox During Pregnancy

- Chicken pox is extremely contagious.
- People may pass the infection for several weeks before they know they have it.
- Avoid anyone with chicken pox until *all* their pox have crusted over.
- If you are exposed or think that you were exposed, call your doctor immediately (weekends included).
- Get vaccinated *before* you get pregnant.
- Most women who think they *haven't* had chicken pox actually *have*. Know your risk. If you don't remember having chicken pox, get tested by your doctor before you get pregnant. A simple blood test can determine whether you've had chicken pox.
- If you had chicken pox before you were pregnant, you can't get it again or pass it to your fetus.
- If you are exposed, consider getting *varicella zoster immune globulin* (VZIG). It's safe and lowers your risk of getting chicken pox. Also, getting VZIG soon after exposure reduces your baby's risk of problems.
- Confirm with the person giving your injection that it's VZIG and not vari-cella *vaccine*. The vaccine should never be used while you're pregnant.
- Ultrasound cannot detect many signs of chicken pox in a fetus.

and other complications as well. If a pregnant woman develops the rare complication of pneumonia with chicken pox, she should be treated in the hospital with IV antiviral drugs.

Q: *I'm a teacher and have heard about something called "fifth disease" among children. I've also heard that I can pass this disease to my fetus if someone in my classroom has it. Is this true?*

A: If you have never had fifth disease and you get it during pregnancy, you may indeed pass it to your fetus, but serious problems are extremely rare.

Fifth disease, also called *erythema infectiosum*, is caused by par-vovirus B19. Parvovirus infection is one of the few that can be transmitted from a mother to her unborn child. Fifth disease is one in a series of six common childhood illnesses that causes rashes. It's a very common viral infection and most commonly passed among children five to fourteen years of age. Infection rates vary seasonally but are higher in winter and spring. In children, the symptoms usually begin with a low-grade fever and general achiness followed a few days later by a rash on the cheeks that spreads to the body and limbs.

Unfortunately, the typical rash appears about five days *after* the virus has disappeared from the bloodstream. In other words, children are most infectious *before* they develop any signs or symptoms of the illness, making it impossible to avoid exposure if you are around children five to fourteen years old.

So what should you do? First, consider that about half of all adults are immune to this illness because they were infected during childhood. People generally don't have a recollection of having this illness, so if you will be around children frequently during the early part of your pregnancy, you should consider getting an antibody test for past exposure to parvovirus B19. A positive test (showing you were exposed in the past) means you don't need to be concerned about exposure during pregnancy.

If you are among the fifty percent of women who are not immune, you need to think about whether it's worth trying to reduce your risk of exposure to parvovirus. Generally, avoiding all children is too hard, particularly because the risk of having a child affected by parvovirus is so small. But only you can make this decision.

If you get parvovirus during the first half of pregnancy, your baby has a fifteen percent chance of infection. This rises to about thirty-five percent if infection occurs in the second half of pregnancy. If your baby does get infected, bad consequences are rare. About two in 100 babies with parvovirus have anything worse than temporary physical problems.

Q: *My friend's son was over yesterday and today I heard that he has parvovirus. What should I do?*

A: If you are exposed to parvovirus and know or suspect that you have not had the infection in the past, you should call your obstetrician. He or she may recommend testing you and if you are at risk (have never had parvovirus), doing an ultrasound to try to determine if your baby is developing an infection. Sometimes, ultrasound can identify signs of infection but in other cases, more invasive testing (like fetal blood testing) may be necessary. Because the chance of serious injury to the fetus from parvovirus is so low, your doctor probably won't recommend any intervention unless there is strong evidence that your baby has a severe infection.

This viral infection very rarely causes complications in pregnancy so it's not something to worry too much about. Doctors don't recommend testing women for parvovirus when they get pregnant because the infection is so unlikely to cause problems.

Children can spread parvovirus before they develop any outward signs of the illness. And most pregnant women are around children at some point, so avoiding exposure just isn't possible. Your best defense against parvovirus is plain old luck.

Q: *My cat has parvovirus and I want to give her to a friend for the remainder of my pregnancy. Is this a good idea?*

A: If you don't like cats, it's a great idea. But if you're doing it to reduce your risk of catching parvovirus, it's not. Only *human* parvovirus B19 has been linked to fetal problems. Dogs or cats that have parvovirus cannot transmit it to humans, nor can humans give their infections to animals.

Q: *I had a fever in early pregnancy. Is it true that this can cause brain damage in my unborn child?*

A: No, it's not, but I can tell you where this idea got started. There is a relatively rare group of birth defects called neural tube defects. In one out of every 1,000 babies, the spine or back of the skull do not form normally. You can reduce the already low risk by taking a folate supplement during early pregnancy (or by getting at least 400 micrograms of folic acid in your diet). (This is discussed in greater detail in Chapter 4.) Fevers of greater than 102 degrees during the first six weeks of pregnancy (when the spinal cord and skull are normally forming) are associated with a slightly increased risk of neural tube defects.

What's unclear is whether it's the infection or the resulting fever that increases the risk. That is, it may be that certain types of infection raise the risk of neural tube defects and these infections also cause fever. Or it may be that fevers above 102 degrees by themselves raise the risk.

Because no one knows the answer, many doctors recommend that women with fevers during the first six weeks of pregnancy take Tylenol to reduce their body temperature. In fact, there is no evidence that holding your fever down with medications reduces your risk of neural tube defects. In other words, even though fever and increased risk of neural tube defects have been linked, it is not clear that you can separate this linkage by reducing your body temperature.

Only temperatures of greater than 102 degrees have been linked with this small increased risk. If your temperature is less than 102 degrees, there is no cause for concern. If it's 103 degrees, I say take the Tylenol. You will almost certainly *feel* better—if it doesn't do anything for your baby.

Q: *What is CMV and can it affect my pregnancy or my baby?*

A: CMV, or *cytomegalovirus,* is a virus in the same family as herpes. People can only get CMV from close contact with an infected person. Most CMV infections come from sexual contact, but CMV can be found in urine or saliva as well. Day care workers are at risk of CMV as it can be passed from a child to a caregiver during diaper changing. Even though you may never have heard of it, between fifty and eighty percent of adults in the United States have had CMV infection. Usually, it produces no symptoms at all. As with the other herpes viruses, once cytomegalovirus infects a person, it remains in her body for life. The virus generally lies dormant and does not cause any serious problems.

If you get your first CMV infection during pregnancy, your baby has a thirty to forty percent risk of infection. Of babies infected in utero, fewer than one in ten has any lasting consequences. Hearing loss is the most common severe consequence of congenital infection. A baby infected in utero cannot be treated. The *mother* can sometimes be treated, but the drugs may be riskier than the infection itself.

If you've had CMV infections in the past, you may, at some point, develop a "reactivation" infection, meaning the "sleeping" virus reawakens, which also causes few symptoms. In one out of 1,000 reactivation infections in pregnant women, the baby will develop an infection as well. But CMV infection is one of the many unavoidable risks in pregnancy.

There is no sure way to prevent infection, nor is there any proven treatment, but you can reduce your risk of getting a primary CMV infection. If you are sexually active and not monogamous, use condoms. (Although the virus may still be transmitted in the saliva, condom use will decrease your risk.) Washing your hands after changing diapers or coming into contact with any bodily fluids (urine, saliva, feces) will also reduce your risk of getting CMV.

Q: *If I have CMV infection, can I breast-feed?*

A: Absolutely. Breast-feeding has a number of well-demonstrated benefits (including reducing ear infections and allergies). The benefits of breast-feeding almost certainly outweigh the extremely small risk of passing CMV infection through your breast milk.

Q: *I've just had my second urinary tract infection during this pregnancy. Why did this happen, and what can I do to stop it from happening again?*

A: Some women are just more susceptible than others to urinary tract infections. These women have a slight difference in the shape of the cells that line the urinary tract. This subtle difference helps bacteria gain a foothold and begin to multiply—the beginnings of an infection. The "urinary tract," which includes the kidneys, which produce urine; the ureters, which carry urine from the kidneys to the bladder; and the bladder itself, also undergoes changes during pregnancy that make infections more likely, even among women who never got them before pregnancy.

Everyone has thousands of bacteria all over the outside of their bodies. From time to time, small numbers of these bacteria get into the bladder. The body usually either kills these bacteria or holds their numbers in check with its own natural defense mechanisms. If the bacteria increase in number, they cause the burning, urge to urinate, and need to urinate frequently that are the most common symptoms of a bladder infection.

After infecting the bladder, the bacteria can move upward through the ureters and infect the kidneys. Bladder infections themselves are annoying, but kidney infections can be downright dangerous, leading to kidney damage if not treated.

Several bodily changes increase your chance of getting a urinary tract infection during pregnancy. First, the bladder may not empty completely because it's compressed by the uterus. The small amount of urine remaining in the bladder provides a breeding ground for any bacteria that are already there.

During pregnancy, the ureters function slightly differently than when you're not pregnant. They relax somewhat, allowing urine to pass from the bladder back up toward the kidneys instead of only flowing *away* from the kidneys. The ureters may also be compressed as pregnancy progresses, slowing the normal flow of urine out of the kidneys. This allows an infection that begins in the bladder to move more easily up to the kidneys.

Not only are bladder infections more common during pregnancy, they're more dangerous as well, since bladder infections can cause preterm contractions. One of the things your health care provider does at almost every prenatal visit is to perform a simple "dipstick" test of your urine. This test looks for early signs of a bladder infection. If the signs are there (in the form of protein or other substances in the urine) your provider will probably want to treat you with antibiotics, even if you don't have any symptoms, to prevent things from getting worse. When you're not pregnant, these early warning signs are usually not treated, since your body fights most early infections on its own.

Luckily, treating urinary tract infections is simple and safe during pregnancy. Your doctor will probably prescribe a seven-to-ten-day course of one of several antibiotics known to be safe and effective in pregnancy (see page 62 for a list of some of these). Doctors prefer giving at least a week of antibiotics, rather than the shorter courses used outside of pregnancy, to reduce the chance of the infection returning.

When you're not pregnant, drinking pure cranberry juice daily can reduce your risk of infection, but no studies show that it can be used to treat infections during pregnancy. Because of the potentially serious consequences of an untreated infection, and the lack of evidence that cranberry juice helps, I recommend sticking to antibiotics to treat bladder infections during pregnancy.

If you're unlucky enough to have more than one urinary tract infection during pregnancy, your doctor should probably give you "prophylactic" antibiotics every day. This means you take a low dose of antibiotics (usually one-fourth or less of the usual dose) once a day. Prophylactic treatment reduces the risk of recurrent infection, and only antibiotics that are safe in pregnancy would be used. Other than taking this daily dose of antibiotics, there isn't much to be done to prevent recurrence. Many doctors recommend drinking lots of water or cranberry juice, but these interventions should only be used in combination with, not instead of, antibiotics.

Q: *Why have I had so many yeast infections during my pregnancy?*

A: Researchers think the hormones released during pregnancy change the normal chemical makeup of the vagina, making a yeast infection more likely. Most people, men and women, pregnant or not, have some yeast (technically called candida) growing in or on their bodies. Often the yeast lives in the digestive tract and in the vagina—even when there are no symptoms. Some studies show that for every woman who complains about a yeast infection or vaginal discharge, four more have yeast growing in the vagina and don't have any symptoms.

Pregnant women are more prone to yeast infections, but these infections can't hurt the baby at all. You should treat the infection if it is bothersome, and ignore it if it's not. Vaginal yeast infections don't increase the risk of preterm labor or cause any other pregnancy-related problems.

Treatment during pregnancy is exactly the same as outside of pregnancy—vaginal creams or pills—and both work equally well. The most common pill, fluconazole (Diflucan), has been studied in pregnancy and does not cause any harm to the baby. Vaginal creams (such as miconazole or terconazole) are also safe during pregnancy—they are usually given for a full seven to ten days in pregnancy, rather than the three days sometimes recommended to nonpregnant women, which can lower the failure rate of this treatment.

Q: *What's the difference between gestational diabetes and regular diabetes? Does having one mean I will definitely have the other?*

A: There are three kinds of diabetes. People with Type 1 diabetes do not make any insulin and need daily insulin injections or they will die. Type 2 diabetics make insulin but their bodies are resistant to it. Type 2 diabetics usually manage their diabetes by taking pills rather than insulin injections. Gestational diabetes (sometimes called Type 3 diabetes) is similar to Type 2 diabetes. The body makes insulin but the placenta makes a hormone (human placental lactogen) that counteracts insulin, making the woman resistant to her own insulin during pregnancy. Treatment involves diet changes (lowering the amount of simple sugar in the diet), diet, and sometimes insulin.

If you have Type 1 or Type 2 diabetes before pregnancy, you will definitely have it during pregnancy. In either case, you should discuss your condition with your obstetrician *before* you get pregnant. Women who have good control of their diabetes before they get pregnant are much less likely to suffer complications during pregnancy.

If you have gestational diabetes, you have a higher risk of developing Type 2 diabetes in the future. Women with gestational diabetes have about a one in three chance of developing diabetes at some point in their lives. For this reason, if you have been diagnosed with gestational diabetes, you should have annual screening for diabetes (possibly for the rest of your life).

Q: *I have Type 2 diabetes (I control it with medication). What do I have to worry about during my pregnancy?*

A: Your biggest concern during pregnancy should be maintaining good control of your blood sugar, just like before pregnancy. Good blood sugar control protects your baby from harm. If blood sugar levels are too high during the first six to eight weeks of pregnancy, the baby's heart may not develop normally. Diabetic women should always seek a doctor's care *before* they try to get pregnant, and try to normalize their blood sugar levels as much as possible for several months before getting pregnant.

During pregnancy, doctors prefer to treat Type 2 diabetes with insulin rather than oral medication, as early studies linked oral diabetes medication with birth defects. The latest evidence suggests that oral medications may in fact be safe. But until there are more studies, these medications won't be the standard treatment. For now, even if you're used to taking pills to control your diabetes, you might have to take insulin injections during pregnancy.

Q: *Do gestational diabetes and Type 2 diabetes pose the same risks to my baby?*

A: No, not at all. Gestational diabetes has very few ill effects for the baby, even if left untreated. Women with gestational diabetes tend to have more cesarean deliveries and bigger babies (called "macrosomic" babies—which just means bigger). These bigger babies may also have some mild abnormalities in blood chemistry at birth. These abnormalities resolve quickly and do not cause lasting harm. Treatment of gestational diabetes lowers the chance of macrosomia, but not the rate of cesarean delivery or other birth complications. Women with gestational diabetes do not have an increased risk of cardiac or other birth defects.

Q: *Why is there so much difference between the risks of gestational and non-gestational diabetes?*

A: The fetal organs develop between weeks two and twelve, and only during this time can high blood sugar cause birth defects. Since gesta-

Diabetes in Pregnancy

Type of diabetes	Usual treatment in pregnancy	Risks of poor control
Type 1 or juvenile onset	Continue insulin	Mother: kidney damage, blindness, coma, death Baby: birth defects, poor growth
Type 2 or adult onset	Diet, exercise, stop pills for diabetes and change to insulin*	Mother: kidney damage, blindness, increased cesarean risk Baby: birth defects, excess growth
Type 3 or gestational	Diet, exercise, insulin	Mother: increased cesarean risk Baby: excess growth

*Some doctors are beginning to use pills to control Type 2 and 3 diabetes, but it's not common practice.

tional diabetics have *normal* blood sugar during the early part of their pregnancy (it only rises after the middle of pregnancy), they do not face these risks. Obstetricians test for gestational diabetes at about twenty-six weeks of pregnancy. Treatment of blood sugar after twenty-six weeks can't affect organ development since organs are fully formed. Testing for gestational diabetes is aimed instead at reducing the cesarean delivery rate. Gestational diabetics tend to have big babies. Big babies mean more cesareans.

This does not mean gestational diabetes needn't be taken seriously, but simply that the consequences of pregestational diabetes and gestational diabetes are very different. Obstetricians treat gestational diabetes with diet modification and exercise. If these treatments fail, doctors recommend insulin. In most cases, gestational diabetes resolves shortly after delivery. Gestational diabetics have an increased risk of developing diabetes later in life, so you should get tested for Type 2 diabetes annually if you've had gestational diabetes.

Q: *My husband says I should stop taking my blood pressure medication while I'm pregnant because it could hurt the baby. What do you think?*

A: Your husband may be right, but you need to discuss your situation with your doctor before doing anything. Hypertension, or high blood pressure, affects millions of Americans and is becoming more common.

Over the long run (meaning more than ten years), even minor elevations of blood pressure can increase the risk of heart attacks and strokes. Untreated high blood pressure may be responsible for almost 50,000 deaths a year in the United States alone. Understandably, doctors have become much more aggressive about treating high blood pressure.

In pregnancy, things may be different. Hypertensive pregnant women do face higher risks of complications, but taking blood pressure medication won't eliminate these risks. Sound a bit confusing? Problems from high blood pressure develop very slowly (decades or more) while pregnancy lasts less than a year (although it may not seem like it). Most of the usual problems of high blood pressure won't show up in this short period of time, making treatment less useful. In addition, some blood pressure medications can actually be bad for the developing baby.

Deciding whether blood pressure medication should be continued or stopped during pregnancy requires a bit of thought. Pregnant women with very high blood pressure (when the lower number, or diastolic pressure, is greater than 110) should definitely be treated during pregnancy. Blood pressure this high can cause dangerous complications, even in the short run. For pregnant women with blood pressure between 120/80 and 200/110, it's not clear whether medication should be continued. Some medications appear safe while others do not. Because of these complexities, if you have elevated blood pressure, you should get the advice of an obstetrician trained in caring for high-risk pregnancies before deciding what to do.

Q: *I have asthma and I don't want to use my inhaler too much because I'm afraid of its effect on my baby. What should I do?*

A: You should stop worrying about your baby getting too much medication and start worrying about your baby getting enough oxygen. The air passages in an asthmatic's lungs begin to close in response to irritation when other peoples' lungs would simply ignore the irritant. Closing these airways can reduce the amount of oxygen in the bloodstream. Reducing the baby's oxygen level can be *extremely* dangerous, causing growth delay and other serious developmental problems.

Doctors and patients *undertreat* asthma much more than they *overtreat* it. Numerous studies have shown that people usually use too little medication, not too much. The consequences of untreated asthma are much worse than any potential side effects of asthma medications. Reducing your medications because you're pregnant is clearly a *bad* idea.

The best way to treat asthma during pregnancy is to take enough medication so that you don't even have asthma attacks. Treating yourself only when you have wheezing may be exactly the opposite of what you should do. Anybody who uses a short-acting inhaler (like albuterol) more than twice a week would be better off on a daily steroid inhaler instead. These powerful drugs reduce asthma complications even better than do the typical short-acting inhalers and have no adverse effects on pregnancy. In fact, well-done scientific studies of asthma drugs have shown they are safe in pregnancy.

Do yourself and your baby a favor and get enough oxygen. Take your medicine.

Q: *I want to change from my prescription antidepressant to St. John's Wort. It must be safer since it's natural, right?*

A: "Natural" doesn't mean better or safer. A drug strong enough to help you is strong enough to hurt you, so if St. John's Wort can cure your depression, it might be able to cause problems as well. I'm a big fan of natural and herbal medications in many circumstances, but not in this case. St. John's Wort can be an effective treatment for depression but has not been well studied in pregnancy. In fact, Prozac has a much better safety record in pregnancy than St. John's Wort. I don't recommend St. John's Wort during pregnancy.

Q: *I have depression and was on Prozac for a long time. If I quit when I'm pregnant, I'm afraid that I might become depressed. If I stay on it, I'm worried about the baby. What should I do?*

A: First, you should do nothing without talking to your psychiatrist or therapist. Depression is a serious illness and may require treatment throughout pregnancy. You and your doctor must carefully weigh the risks and benefits of treatment. In this case, the benefits are obvious: You feel better, and you're not depressed. So, what are the risks? In one study, minor birth defects (those that don't require surgery or impair a child's function) were slightly increased in women who took Prozac. A much larger study of more than 2,000 women has found no signs of harm. The results from the larger study are much more important than those from the smaller one. Small studies are more prone to error since their findings are more likely to result from chance alone. Simply stated, Prozac poses no identifiable risks to your baby.

Q: *Well, what about the effects of Prozac on the child after birth?*

A: Several small studies of children age six to seven who were exposed to Prozac prenatally showed no ill effects. However, these were very small studies and more information is needed. The key is weighing the risks and benefits. Stopping antidepressants could be much worse than being on them. It might seem obvious, but if you die your baby can't possibly survive. Even less drastic effects of depression, like not caring for your baby well, can be more harmful that the medicines used to treat depression are. If you are depressed, a safe antidepressant like Prozac might be the best possible thing for you.

Similarly, you will probably be able to continue the Prozac while you breast-feed. Some babies develop vomiting and diarrhea if their mothers take Prozac while breast-feeding. These problems are common and the symptoms will stop when the drug is stopped. You must weigh these potential problems against the larger benefit you get from taking the medication. Changing antidepressants is not something to take lightly. But if any problems develop, you can discuss a medication change with your obstetrician, pediatrician, and psychiatrist.

Q: *I have obsessive/compulsive disorder and I take Paxil. Is this dangerous during pregnancy?*

A: It doesn't appear to be. There are studies of hundreds of babies born to women who took Paxil during pregnancy and they had no more birth defects than would be expected (about three percent of the babies had some type of birth defect). Women who took Paxil during pregnancy had no more miscarriages than those who didn't take it. And Paxil does not appear to impair fertility. On the other hand, reports of 200 to 300 women who have done well taking Paxil isn't enough to say it's completely safe. Studies of thousands of women may be needed to be sure there are no rare adverse effects.

Talk to your obstetrician and the doctor who treats your OCD. Your decision whether or not to stay on the drug should depend on your level of impairment off the drug. In other words, you must weigh the risks and benefits. In this case, you have to carefully consider the known benefit (relief of symptoms) against some unknown, probably small, risk.

Q: *I was diagnosed with breast cancer last year. I seem to be completely healthy now and I want to get pregnant. Is there any reason I should wait?*

A: This question can only be answered in consultation with the doctor who treated you for your breast cancer, since there are probably many clinical details that are specific only to you. On the whole, however, getting pregnant after having breast cancer doesn't change your chance of having a recurrence. In fact, some new evidence suggests that women with breast cancer who get pregnant shortly afterward have a *better* outcome than those who don't. I wouldn't suggest getting pregnant to reduce your recurrence risk, but I would say that you needn't worry about getting pregnant.

> ### Staying Healthy During Pregnancy
>
> - Wash hands frequently to avoid colds
> - Get a flu shot, particularly if you'll be in the second or third trimester during flu season (November to March)
> - Don't stop your medications without talking to your doctor

Treating breast cancer *during* pregnancy can be complicated. Most breast cancer specialists prefer women to wait several years after treatment before getting pregnant. This simplifies the doctor's life since it's difficult to manage a recurrence during pregnancy. It can be done, however. If you have important personal reasons for wanting to get pregnant soon after your initial treatment, you should consider it. It won't worsen your prognosis. By the same token, if you get pregnant by accident, don't have an abortion in the hopes that it will lower your recurrence risk. Studies have shown that it won't.

8 You Know You Shouldn't:

Everything You Need to Know About
Cigarettes, Alcohol, and Drugs

"There is more refreshment and stimulation in a nap, even of the briefest, than in all the alcohol ever distilled."—Ovid

Cigarettes, alcohol, and illicit drugs are bad for you—cigarettes cause cancer, alcohol can impair your judgment, and other drugs are addictive, illegal, or both—but will they harm your baby? Surprisingly, some will and some may not. Our society tends to take an all-or-none approach to these substances. Yet research shows that alcohol in small amounts appears safe. You may choose to avoid all alcohol during pregnancy, but if you don't want to abstain completely, this chapter helps you understand how to gauge whether your intake is safe or not. This chapter also addresses the risks of smoking during pregnancy and gives some advice on ways to quit.

Q: *My mother smoked while she was pregnant with me. Why should I stop smoking during my pregnancy?*

A: You should stop smoking because it's bad for you whether you are pregnant or not. Cigarette smoke contains an incredibly diverse number of toxic substances. Smoking is probably the single largest cause of preventable illness in the United States. (In a book devoted to what you *can*

do during pregnancy, you might be surprised that there a few things you *can't* do. But smoking is definitely one of these things.)

Smoking cigarettes makes it harder to get pregnant whether naturally or using technologies like in vitro fertilization. Smoking also increases the risk of miscarriage. Men who smoke have slightly lower sperm quality (but this does not seem to lower pregnancy rates).

Cigarette smoking during pregnancy slows fetal growth, increases the risk of prematurity, increases the risk of placenta previa (in which the placenta grows over the opening through which the baby has to pass to be born), and increases the risk that the baby will suffer sudden infant death. Do not smoke.

Q: *I only smoke a few cigarettes. Could that possibly hurt?*

A: Yes. The Surgeon General considers cigarette smoking to be as addictive as heroin and cocaine. Most people who smoke even a few cigarettes do become addicted. Even if you never go beyond smoking just a few cigarettes, you are still putting your baby at risk. Studies show that smoking less than half a pack a day increases your risk of preterm delivery. But smoking less is better than smoking more, so if you can't quit, at least cut down as much as possible.

Q: *I want to quit smoking but my doctor says I have to go cold turkey. Can you give me any advice?*

A: Yes. It's easy to see why your doctor is concerned about giving you nicotine replacement treatment (like Nicorette gum or nicotine patches) during pregnancy. The FDA labels these drugs as "pregnancy category D," meaning they may harm a fetus. This label makes doctors reluctant to prescribe nicotine replacement products to pregnant women. These doctors may not notice that the FDA label also says "the potential benefits may warrant the use of the drug in pregnant women despite the risks."

Replacing cigarette smoking with a patch or gum probably helps the fetus in many ways. Cigarette smoke contains thousands of different compounds, including carbon monoxide, cyanide, nicotine, and tar.

While nicotine patch or gum systems continue to deliver nicotine to a pregnant woman, they remove the risk associated with the thousands of other parts of cigarette smoke.

Cigarette smoking increases the amount of carbon monoxide in the mother's bloodstream. Carbon monoxide keeps the fetus from getting enough oxygen. Replacing cigarette smoke with a nicotine patch decreases carbon monoxide and allows the fetus to get more oxygen. So while nicotine patch or gum users continue to get nicotine, they are no longer being exposed to the other harmful substances in smoke.

I definitely recommend using a nicotine patch or gum if it helps you quit. Quitting smoking is probably the single best thing you will be able to do for yourself and your fetus. Keep trying until you can quit for good.

Q: *I'm around people who smoke, can this affect my pregnancy?*

A: The answer depends on how much they smoke and how much you are around them. Recent studies have shown that passive smoking exposes the fetus to many of the same chemicals that come from active smoking, but at far lower levels. While cigarette smoking can clearly harm a fetus, passive smoking has not been shown to do so. Indeed, research suggests that if environmental tobacco smoke does affect a fetus, the effect is very small.

The first real evidence that environmental tobacco smoke reaches the unborn child came from a study measuring nicotine in fetal hair at birth. Since hair in the fetus grows primarily in the third trimester, these tests measure the fetus's third trimester exposure to tobacco smoke. Studies show that babies whose mothers did not smoke, but were around smokers, have measurable nicotine levels in their hair. These studies show that nicotine reaches the fetus, but they didn't show that environmental tobacco smoke can hurt the fetus.

Tobacco smoke clearly hurts the smoker. It clearly hurts passive smokers as well. It is much less clear that it can hurt the *fetus* of a passive smoker. I would simply recommend avoiding passive smoke when possible but not worrying about its effects on your baby if exposure is unavoidable. People seem to be fairly receptive to not smoking around pregnant women, so you might simply ask people to stop and see what happens.

Q: *I like to drink wine with dinner. Is it really true that I have to stop during pregnancy? I heard that in France they don't worry about alcohol in pregnancy at all.*

A: You don't really have to stop drinking completely during pregnancy. You just have to understand a little bit of science so you can make an informed decision.

Researchers generally agree that heavy alcohol use (which means more than two drinks a day on a regular basis or at least one episode of drinking five drinks or more) does increase the risk of a rare problem called *fetal alcohol syndrome*. This condition affects about two out of 1,000 babies born in the United States. Among women who chronically abuse alcohol and drink more than ten drinks a day during pregnancy, two-thirds of their babies escape without any apparent ill effects. I point this out not to encourage alcohol abuse but to demonstrate how *resistant* a fetus is to the toxic effects of alcohol.

The Canadian organization Motherisk examined over 500 scientific articles on alcohol and pregnancy published between 1966 (when fetal alcohol syndrome was first described) and the mid-1990s. The Motherisk researchers concluded that there was *no increased risk of fetal malformations in women who had less than two drinks a day during the first trimester.* The fetus develops all its organs during the first trimester, so drinking during this time would be the most dangerous. Since two or fewer drinks a day in the first trimester caused no problems (the time when the fetus is most sensitive to the effects of alcohol), it wouldn't cause problems in the second or third trimesters either. This doesn't "prove" the safety of moderate alcohol consumption but it does set some limits on the risk. If drinking less than two drinks per day is dangerous, the danger is so small that studies involving more than 100,000 women could not find it.

Medicine is a science and should be based on facts and evidence. The recommendation to completely stop drinking during pregnancy is

Alcohol Equivalency

There are approximately eight grams of absolute alcohol (often considered to be one "unit" or one drink) in each of the following:

- twelve ounces of beer
- one glass of wine
- one shot of hard alcohol
- one small glass of sherry

Drinking more than one drink a day can increase the risk of fetal alcohol syndrome.

not based on fact. The Royal College of Obstetricians and Gynecologists in the UK recommends that pregnant women have no more than one drink per day. U.S. agencies have not taken so enlightened a view, with many U.S. organizations still including statements like "a safe level of alcohol in pregnancy has not been established." While strictly true (no safe level of sunshine has ever been established either by the way), these statements ignore the strong evidence that moderate alcohol use is not dangerous.

You may certainly choose to abstain from all alcohol throughout your pregnancy, but you should do so knowing there is no measurable risk of low-level alcohol consumption. If you want to continue moderate drinking during your pregnancy, you should be reassured that there is no scientific reason to stop. If you live in the United States, you may still feel the stares of your friends and relatives as you lift a glass of chardonnay in your second trimester.

By the way, it's not true that they don't worry about alcohol in pregnancy in France; it's just that in Europe, the attitude tends to be a bit less alarmist than it is in the United States. European doctors *are* concerned about fetal alcohol syndrome, but they seem to understand the difference between dangerous alcohol use and moderate use.

Q: *Is it true that hard liquor is more dangerous than wine or beer when you're pregnant?*

A: No. The form that alcohol comes in makes no difference to your fetus. Alcohol in drinks is rapidly absorbed in your stomach and enters your bloodstream. Your blood alcohol level determines how much alcohol gets to your fetus. Blood alcohol level depends on how much you drink, not what form it takes.

Q: *I don't smoke cigarettes, drink alcohol, or do any other drugs, but I occasionally do smoke marijuana. What effect can this have on my baby?*

A: Surprisingly perhaps, occasional marijuana smoking appears to have no ill effects on the unborn child. Believe me, your friends and relatives will think you're *insane* if you tell them that you smoked marijuana during pregnancy, so if you intend to do it, keep your mouth shut. Don't forget it's illegal.

Most studies of marijuana use and pregnancy have focused on heavy users, usually someone who smokes more than five joints a week. If researchers can't find any effects in heavy smokers, then such effects would be even *less* likely in occasional smokers. There have been literally hundreds of scientific articles looking for adverse effects of marijuana smoking, and many have looked at potential adverse effects of marijuana smoking on pregnancy. The two largest and best designed studies found no association between marijuana use (even heavy use) and miscarriage, complications, or major or minor physical abnormalities. Several small studies have found a connection between the size of the baby and heavy first trimester marijuana use, but this finding has not been consistent. In two large studies, marijuana users had *larger* babies than nonusers (though not by much).

I certainly do not recommend smoking marijuana during pregnancy. On the other hand, I find no evidence that occasional marijuana smoking poses any danger to the unborn child. I say this not to recommend marijuana smoking, but merely to point out that occasional marijuana use appears less dangerous than cigarette smoking.

Q: *If marijuana won't make my baby deformed, premature, or small, will it make him stupid?*

A: There is no evidence that heavy marijuana smoking will lower a child's intelligence. Indeed, in three large studies, marijuana had no effect on IQ scores. This stands in stark contrast to cigarettes: IQ scores drop as a mother's cigarette smoking increases. That is, heavy cigarette smokers consistently have children with lower IQs than do nonsmokers. While marijuana use does not lower overall intelligence, some scientists believe it affects reasoning skills. These suspicious are far from proven.

Q: *What effect can cocaine have on my baby?*

A: Cocaine and cigarettes are two of the most dangerous substances to use in pregnancy. It's difficult to study the effects of cocaine on pregnancy because many women who use cocaine use other drugs as well. So, it's very hard to separate the effects of cocaine from the effects of these other drugs. However, Dr. Gideon Koren and colleagues at the Hospital for Sick Children in Toronto examined over 600 scientific studies on prenatal cocaine use. Their report suggests that cocaine remains one of the most dangerous drugs used in pregnancy.

In general, the risk of having a child with a major birth defect is about one percent. This risk nearly doubled if the mother used cocaine during pregnancy. Similarly, while five to ten percent of non-cocaine users have babies weighing less than 2,500 grams, this risk was almost three times as high if the mother used cocaine during her pregnancy. Babies born to mothers who use are more likely to be premature. Mothers who use cocaine have an increased risk for a condition called *abruptio placenta,* in which the placenta rapidly tears away from the uterine wall, potentially killing the fetus.

Cocaine affects pregnancy in a way similar to cigarettes. Both drugs constrict blood vessels and reduce blood flow to the placenta.

Substance Use and Pregnancy

- Smoking cigarettes lowers birth weight and increases the risk of prematurity
- If you can't quit smoking, cut down—any reduction is better than none
- Drinking more than one drink a day can be dangerous and increases the risk of fetal alcohol syndrome
- Cocaine use can lead to low birth weight, prematurity, and birth defects

Some researchers believe that many things that people see as effects of cocaine are actually effects of tobacco. Almost all cocaine users smoke cigarettes. Though this debate rages in the scientific community, it shows the power of tobacco companies to manipulate the press, since reports of "tobacco babies" don't make the nightly news the way reports of "crack babies" do.

Tobacco smoking during pregnancy is a far greater public health hazard than cocaine use. This may sound unbelievable but consider this: Fewer than one percent of pregnant women use cocaine but as many as twenty percent of pregnant women smoke cigarettes. Even if using cocaine were ten times as bad as cigarette smoking (and it's not clear that it is), tobacco smoke would hurt far more babies.

The bottom line is to stay away from tobacco *and* cocaine, not to choose one over the other.

Q: *Can I be prosecuted for drinking or taking drugs during my pregnancy?*

A: You can be *prosecuted* but you probably can't be convicted—though that would be a small comfort. No court has yet upheld charges of child endangerment, delivering drugs to minors, or child abuse against a mother who used alcohol or drugs while pregnant. All such convictions have been overturned on appeal, with the appellate courts consistently concluding that the laws used to prosecute these mothers were not designed for such a purpose.

Although such prosecutions might seem appealing to some people, they are counterproductive, fail to protect children, and are used in a racist manner. Consider that although white women use drugs during pregnancy just as often as women of color, women of color are usually the target of these charges. More importantly, cigarette smoking causes literally thousands of times more prenatal damage than do illegal drugs, yet you never hear of mothers being charged with child abuse for smoking.

Prosecuting women for their drug problems reflects society's belief that some women (particularly poor women or women of color) just can't make good decisions. Increasing access to drug counseling and treatment during pregnancy would undoubtedly be a far more productive use of energy and funds. The American Academy of Pediatrics, the March of Dimes Foundation, the American Medical Association, and the American Public Health Association all agree that it's a mistake to prosecute pregnant drug users.

9 Exercise For Two:

Staying Fit While Pregnant

Patient: Doctor, can I play basketball while I'm pregnant?
Doctor: Of course.
Patient: That's wonderful, I could never play before!

What kind of exercise can you do during pregnancy? Almost anything you could do before you got pregnant. Doctors recognize that regular, strenuous exercise has many benefits, from reducing the risk of diabetes and cancer to extending life expectancy. But concerns about raising the body temperature, becoming dehydrated, or even causing premature labor have led some doctors to recommend that their pregnant patients stop, or significantly cut back on, their exercise. This chapter addresses these and many other concerns. It reviews the best available research about exercise during pregnancy and reveals that in almost all cases exercise is not only safe, but also can measurably improve the chance of a good outcome from pregnancy. The chapter also addresses some specific dos and don'ts for exercising while pregnant, and gives tips on how to tell when you're at the "right" level of exertion.

Q: *I read that I shouldn't exercise during pregnancy, is that true?*

A: Of course not! Imagine a scene 20,000 years ago: A saber-toothed tiger chases a pregnant woman. If she doesn't run fast enough that's the end of her and her future child. If it really wasn't safe to run in pregnancy, none of our ancestors could have gotten away from those tigers—and that would have meant good-bye human race. Continuing an established exercise program during pregnancy isn't just safe, it's smart. Fit women have shorter, easier labors—and they have a head start when it comes to chasing their babies around! For healthy women there is simply no danger to exercising in pregnancy.

Needless to say, there are risks in any type of exercise, but these risks are completely acceptable with most types of exercise. Of course you'll be worried about protecting your baby, but your body has done a good job of that already. Your body diverts a large amount of blood to your uterus in pregnancy—even when you're exercising. The developing fetus is also protected by its amniotic sac, the wall of the uterus, and your abdominal wall. So short of a car accident or gunshot wound, it's very hard to hurt the baby through all those layers. It certainly seems sensible to limit risky activities like hang gliding or rock climbing during pregnancy, but walking, running, swimming, biking, gardening, tennis, and most other noncontact sports are fine.

Q: *How hard should I work out when I'm pregnant?*

A: Your heart works harder during pregnancy than before, so you should listen to your body. If you normally tire after thirty minutes of walking, you may find that you've had it after twenty now. That's fine. Listen to your body and quit at twenty minutes. You'll build your tolerance back up if you continue. Some people will tell you that exercising harder than a certain amount is dangerous, but the American College of Obstetricians and Gynecologists (ACOG) says "there are no data . . . that pregnant women should limit exercise intensity and lower target heart rates because of potential adverse effects." In addition, the slight increase in body temperature that comes with vigorous exercise has no harmful effects on the developing fetus.

If you want to start a new exercise program during pregnancy, it's a good idea to start slowly—try about ten to twenty minutes of walking on the first day. If you can still carry on a conversation, but feel out of breath, that's probably a good level of activity. If you can't talk, you're working too hard. You don't want to wear yourself out—it will discourage you from continuing with your exercise program. If you can talk easily, you may not be working hard enough. That's OK to start, but as you get comfortable with your activity, you can try to increase your intensity until you're somewhat out of breath as you exercise. For bike riding or swimming, I would say the same thing. Try ten to twenty minutes to start and build slowly, adding five minutes each week. It's also fine to exercise in short bursts—ten minutes three times a day, rather than thirty minutes all at once.

Try to stay well hydrated—drink enough to keep yourself from feeling thirsty. There's no need to drink expensive sports drinks; plain water works just fine. Drinking soda, juice, and sports drinks does make some people feel more energetic during exercise, so feel free to drink these if they seem to help. The idea that you need "electrolytes" or some other special fluids during exercise while pregnant is incorrect. Unless you are vomiting, have severe diarrhea, or are taking diuretic medications (drugs to prevent water retention), your body can adjust its own electrolyte balance perfectly well. All you need to do is drink when you get thirsty.

Q: *At my gym, there are big signs on the sauna and hot tub saying that pregnant women shouldn't use them, why is that?*

A: Studies in people and animals show that raising body temperature beyond the normal range can increase the risk of birth defects. The difficulty is in translating this observation into reasonable advice for pregnant women. How high and for how long does the temperature need to be elevated to cause problems?

There is no simple answer, but there certainly are some safe guidelines. First, remember that the risk of temperature elevation depends on your stage of pregnancy. Exposure before you miss a period won't result in birth defects, since the baby's organ systems do not begin forming until two weeks after conception. Conception usually occurs around the middle of the cycle, so the first missed period is at about two weeks of development.

The most sensitive period for causing birth defects extends from two to nine weeks after conception. If you're counting weeks from your last period (that's how your obstetrician keeps track), the most sensitive time extends from week four to week eleven (see box on page 29 for an explanation of the difference between weeks since conception and weeks of pregnancy).

Studies in animals during this sensitive time show that the body temperature must be at least three or four degrees Fahrenheit above normal to increase the risk of birth defects. For obvious reasons, similar studies can't be done in people, but keeping your body temperature below 102 degrees probably eliminates any risk. The next question, of course, is whether hot tubs or saunas are likely to raise the body temperature above 102 degrees.

The temperature in a sauna may be more than 180 F, while hot tubs generally aren't set higher than 104 F. Yet surprisingly, hot tubs may be more dangerous than saunas for pregnant women, simply because it's your *body* temperature that matters, not the temperature around you.

In the sauna, sweating cools the body down, but you don't sweat in a hot tub. People also tend to spend less time in the sauna than in the hot tub, so if body temperature does go up it may not be elevated long enough to do any damage. The study that started most people worrying about hot tubs in pregnancy came out in 1992. The researchers found no link between saunas and birth defects, although there was such a link with hot tubs. After reading the study, many doctors began to recommend that pregnant women avoid hot tubs *and* saunas, even though the study itself didn't demonstrate a risk. An older study of Finnish women, who sauna regularly, found no risk of short (ten minute or less) repeated saunas throughout pregnancy.

As a result of these and other studies, I recommend limiting your time in the hot tub during pregnancy. When you begin to feel overheated, get out. If the temperature is kept over 102 degrees, don't stay in for more than ten minutes at a stretch, even if you don't feel overheated. A hot bath is safer, since the water temperature usually begins in the nineties and cools as you soak, making it nearly impossible to create dangerous temperature levels.

Saunas appear safer than hot tubs, particularly if you keep your exposure short. Keep your saunas to five or ten minutes, get out if you feel overheated or dizzy, and to be extra cautious avoid either saunas or hot tubs until you've hit twelve weeks.

Q: *I've heard that doing sit-ups (or aerobics where I have to lie on my back) is dangerous in pregnancy, is this true?*

A: While it's true that sit-ups become difficult when the uterus is large, there simply isn't any known danger in doing them. Lying on your back is fine as well—some studies show a decrease in blood supply to the uterus in this position, but a decrease in blood supply is a laboratory finding. It is in no way the same as saying "the baby isn't getting enough blood." Remember, your pregnancy was built to survive the rigors of life. Lying on your back for a few minutes while you do sit-ups isn't going to hurt anything.

The American College of Obstetricians and Gynecologists recommends that you not do prolonged exercise lying on your back after thirteen weeks of pregnancy. They don't define "prolonged," but ten minutes or less is certainly safe—unless you start to feel light-headed lying on your back, in which case common sense says to stop. Anyway, if you're like me, you can only do about ninety seconds worth of sit-ups before you're in total agony.

Q: *I want to continue with yoga during my pregnancy, should I start going to one of those "prenatal" yoga classes, or continue with what I was doing before?*

A: If you are careful, there is no reason you can't continue doing what you were doing before you got pregnant. The joints clearly become more flexible in many women as they progress through pregnancy. The body releases more of the hormone called *relaxin* during pregnancy, and obstetricians have long thought this hormone might be responsible for the increase in joint flexibility seen during pregnancy. Recent research has cast doubt on whether relaxin is completely responsible but, whatever the cause, changes in joint flexibility do occur with pregnancy.

Prenatal yoga instructors may be more aware of the changes in a woman's body during pregnancy. Their classes are designed to accommodate these changes, so these classes might be easier to manage while pregnant. On the other hand, there is no real danger in trying to continue with standard yoga classes. Just pay attention to your body; if something hurts—stop.

Yoga is terrific for you. I've observed that women who do yoga regularly through pregnancy gain less weight and have easier labors than women who don't exercise. So whatever you do, don't give it up during your pregnancy. Furthermore, women who are physically active recover from delivery much more quickly and have fewer aches and pains as well.

Q: *I love skiing, when should I stop?*

A: There is no good answer to this question. Skiing itself is not harmful, of course. The danger is what happens when you fall. Because of the baby's protection behind your abdominal wall and your uterus, and because the baby is suspended in amniotic fluid—which can act as a shock absorber—a fall that's not hard enough to hurt you won't hurt your baby either.

Most pregnant women I've taken care of don't feel comfortable skiing after the first trimester (thirteen weeks). I don't have any way to judge whether skiing is more dangerous than other activities when pregnant—but unless you have the overwhelming urge to get out there and shred, I'd say switch to something else for the remainder of your pregnancy.

Q: *What other sports should I avoid when pregnant?*

A: Well, I think you should definitely give up skydiving by your due date. Seriously, most women have a natural inclination to play it a little safer during pregnancy than at other times and I think that's perfectly normal. The thing to remember is that exercise is good for you. It's good when you're not pregnant, and it's good when you are. Unless you're into an extreme sport like skydiving or bungee jumping, there's usually an alternative to just giving it up.

Bicycling, for example, is something women have been told to avoid late in pregnancy because of the risk that they'll fall and injure their babies. First, as I mentioned before, you generally have to hurt yourself before your baby will be hurt. And if you've logged thousands of miles on the bike without injury, then the odds are in your favor that continuing through pregnancy will be safe. If you get on a bike and don't *feel* off balance, you should be fine. Biking can get tough later in pregnancy when your belly is big, so I would suggest stationary biking as an alternative (you can use rollers or a wind trainer if you like the feel of really biking—look in a bicycling magazine for ideas).

Scuba diving has generally not been considered safe during pregnancy and in the absence of evidence that it is, I would recommend staying on the surface.

Strangely enough, gardening without wearing gloves may be riskier than any of the activities mentioned above. In a study of over 1,000 women in Europe, gardening without gloves led to an increased risk of toxoplasmosis infection (one of the few infections that can hurt a developing fetus), probably because of exposure to cat feces, which are a source of infection. Of course, this study was done in Europe, where risk factors for infection may be different, but it seems believable. Simply wearing gardening gloves and washing your hands after gardening can make this activity safer (for more details see Chapter 7: Sickness and Health, and Chapter 13: Around the House).

Q: *I've been a marathon runner for years. What should I do with my training regimen now that I'm pregnant?*

A: Congratulations on being in such good shape and on getting pregnant. Elite athletes like you have a special set of issues to think about. Usually high intensity athletes have more trouble *getting* pregnant than avoiding problems *during* pregnancy. That's because most women don't ovulate (the ovary doesn't release an egg) when their percent body fat falls below a certain amount. I usually see this problem in young athletes who haven't had periods for a while and wonder why. It seems that the body figures that if there isn't enough fat around to support a pregnancy, why bother trying?

Once you're pregnant, or visibly pregnant anyway—which may be later than in nonathletes—you will get plenty of comments from friends, relatives (particularly mothers-in-law), and other runners about how you ought to stop training. *Don't listen to them.*

Many marathon runners and other highly conditioned athletes will become depressed if they quit exercising (studies of injured athletes have shown this over and over)—and depression is definitely bad for you and your baby. Rigorous studies of marathon runners and other high-intensity athletes during pregnancy show no ill effects from training while pregnant. That's right. No ill effects. Writing in *Medicine and Science in Sports and Exercise,* Clapp and Dickstein showed that compared with when they weren't pregnant, pregnant women doing weight-bearing exercise (like running) got tired faster—meaning that your maximum ability to exercise is reached about ten percent sooner in the first thirteen weeks of pregnancy and about fifty percent sooner by the third trimester. Swimmers and cyclers (these are considered non-weight-bearing exercise) had a much smaller decrease in exercise intensity. The same authors also found that high-intensity athletes had slightly smaller babies (by about eight ounces), but that the babies were healthy.

Q: *I want to play it safe, why shouldn't I just give up exercise for a few months?*

A: Giving up exercise isn't playing it safe. Inactivity is dangerous for more than one reason. First, your muscles get weak and you're more prone to injury and pain if you are inactive. Second, mothers who are highly conditioned generally have shorter labors by up to several hours and require less pain medication. It only makes sense if you think about it: Who can better handle twenty hours of intense muscular activity by the uterus, someone who mostly watches television or someone who exercises five hours a week?

There are three commonly mentioned reasons for stopping your exercise program during pregnancy: 1) Your baby won't get enough oxygen—it will all go to your muscles, 2) your body temperature will go so high that you'll hurt the baby, and 3) you'll go into preterm labor if you're too active (we all know women who are on bed rest to reduce the risk of preterm labor). Let's go through these one at a time. First, blood flow to the uterus may be slightly reduced during exercise. But a fit heart pumps more efficiently during the twenty-three hours that you're not exercising, which should more than make up for any reduction during exercise.

As to the second point, it's true that body temperature rises during exercise. It's also true that in animals, exposure to high temperatures early in pregnancy can cause birth defects. But studies of humans during pregnancy have failed to show any dangerous temperature rise from exercise. The body does something called "thermoregulation," which is a fancy word for "adjusting to changes in temperature." This means that although you get hot when you exercise, your core body temperature (the temperature your baby is exposed to) doesn't change very much. It certainly stays below 102.5 Fahrenheit (39.2 Celsius), and that's the level at which the fetus is *theoretically* in danger (see Chapter 7 for a discussion of what happens when your temperature goes up from a fever). Furthermore, studies done in the 1980s of women who exercise during pregnancy show that these women *are not* in greater danger of having babies with birth defects.

Finally, increased exercise has *never* been reliably associated with preterm delivery. There are some studies showing that women in jobs that require prolonged standing (like nurses) or work in high-stress settings deliver their babies earlier. But these studies don't apply to voluntary, regular physical activity. Exercise reduces stress hormone levels in your body, so it's not at all the same as working in a stress-filled job. In fact, one study showed that women who exercised regularly were slightly *less* likely to have preterm deliveries.

Q: *What is the gap that women get between the stomach muscles during pregnancy? How can I prevent it from happening?*

A: That "gap" is called the *rectus diastasis*. This fancy Latin phrase means "the gap between the stomach muscles." In truth, there is no "gap." The stomach muscles are joined in the midline by a strong sheet of tissue. This tissue stretches during pregnancy so that there is a wider space between the muscles. In other words, the tissue doesn't disappear but stretches out and then gradually shrinks after delivery. About twenty-five percent of women develop this gap by the second trimester, and the majority of women have it by the third trimester. The rectus diastasis remains for four or five months after delivery in as many as thirty percent of women.

Many popular pregnancy books tell women not to do sit-ups during pregnancy because it will increase the gap. Not only is there no evidence to support this claim, some research shows that women who exercise regularly *before* they get pregnant have a much lower risk of developing a large rectus gap. In any case, the rectus diastasis is a normal part of pregnancy. It allows the uterus to expand without putting excessive strain on the abdominal muscles.

How does this gap develop? Nobody knows, but secretion of the hormone called *relaxin* increases during pregnancy. This hormone allows certain structures in the body to soften and stretch. No scientific studies have demonstrated whether women who have a wider gap in the rectus muscles have more relaxin present or not, but they may. After you deliver, doing abdominal exercise may help shrink the diastasis.

Healthy Pregnancy Tips

Maintain a moderate activity level during pregnancy.

Incorporate warm-up, cool-down, and stretching into your exercise plan.

Stay well hydrated while you exercise.

Be careful when doing activities that present a risk of falling.

If you have medical problems, or haven't exercised before, talk to your doctor before starting an exercise program.

Don't exercise if:
- ❑ your bag of waters has broken
- ❑ you've been treated for preterm labor
- ❑ your baby is not growing normally (your doctor will tell you if this is happening)
- ❑ you are having vaginal bleeding

10 What Is Happening to My Body?

Aches, Pains, and Other Changes

"The body has a mind of its own."—Mason Cooley

Swollen feet, backaches, heartburn, and other aches and pains can turn a healthy pregnancy into a source of discomfort and anxiety. Not only do women suffer from these and other problems more frequently when pregnant than at other times, they face the added problem of wondering whether the treatments they've relied on in the past are safe. The simple act of reaching into the medicine cabinet for Tylenol can provoke mental anguish in many pregnant women. This chapter addresses the bodily changes that many women experience during pregnancy, explains why they happen and how to manage them. After reading this chapter, women will feel comfortable trying some simple lifestyle modifications as well as reaching for a variety of safe over-the-counter medications to treat these common problems.

Q: *What medicines can I take for pain? Is Tylenol the only one that's safe?*

A: You can safely take just about any over-the-counter medication for your pain. Many doctors (and most pregnancy books) say that Tylenol (acetaminophen) is the only safe pain reliever in pregnancy, but there is no reason to be so restrictive. Tylenol is safe, so this drug is worth trying. On the other hand, there is not one bit of evidence linking either aspirin or ibuprofen (Motrin or Advil) with any bad pregnancy outcomes. In fact, some of the best known specialists in high-risk pregnancies believe that aspirin reduces the risk of *preeclampsia* (or high blood pressure in pregnancy). Thousands of women have taken aspirin for this reason without any adverse effects on their babies.

Q: *How can you be so sure these medicines are safe?*

A: The strongest reason to avoid a drug during pregnancy is if it has been proven to be dangerous and has no benefit. For example, Thalidomide should never be used in pregnancy. It causes serious limb deformities in babies of mothers who take it. There are no reasons to take Thalidomide during pregnancy that would outweigh the potential risk to the baby.

For many medications, there may be theoretical reasons to avoid the drugs, but no evidence exists one way or another about their safety. For these drugs, if a safe alternative exists, it might be reasonable to use it. If no safe alternative exists and the drug is necessary, then it probably makes sense to take it. For example, at high doses, the antibiotic gentamicin could theoretically damage a baby's hearing (although it has never been proved to do this). If you have a serious infection, taking gentamicin might be the smartest thing you can do, since the real benefit outweighs the theoretical risk.

Finally, there are drugs that have been studied in pregnancy and have not been found to cause any problems. Technically, it's *never* possible to say that something is completely safe. For example, if scientists study a particular drug during 1,000 pregnancies and don't see any problems, they can only say that problems happen in less than one in every 1,000 pregnancies. They *cannot* say that the drug is 100 percent safe. A recent study found an increased risk of cancer among postmenopausal women who took hormone replacement therapy, but tens of thousands of women were studied before this risk was seen. Breast cancer occurred in about six out of 10,000 women. A study of 1,000 women would not have found this problem.

Aspirin has been studied in thousands of pregnant women without seeing any adverse effects. Theoretically, aspirin and ibuprofen could interfere with the development of the fetal heart. There is no scientific evidence that this actually *occurs;* it's just a theory. In fact, there is evidence that it *does not occur.*

Motherisk (www.motherisk.org), a research organization dedicated to collecting the best available information about drug risk in pregnancy, agrees that aspirin or ibuprofen can be safely taken. If the best drug for the job is aspirin or ibuprofen, it should be taken. If a woman must take high doses for a prolonged period, doctors can use ultrasound to examine the baby and make sure its circulation is normal. If there are signs of developing problems, the drug treatment can be stopped and the abnormalities will disappear. Remember, these drugs do not cause birth defects. Any effects that they might have would be temporary.

It does make sense to avoid aspirin, ibuprofen, and similar drugs at the very end of pregnancy. These drugs interfere with blood clotting and can result in slightly (a few more tablespoons) higher blood loss if you need a cesarean section. They will *not* result in a massive hemorrhage.

Q: *I have terrible heartburn. What can I do about it?*

A: You can treat this common problem with changes in behavior, calcium-containing antacids, and acid-suppressant drugs.

The stomach seems to produce more fluid than usual in early pregnancy and the muscles of the throat, stomach, and intestine are all somewhat more relaxed during pregnancy. Early in pregnancy, these changes can lead to an increased feeling of burning in the stomach or throat. Later in pregnancy, pressure from the developing fetus on the stomach can worsen these symptoms.

Eating smaller meals and not lying down immediately after eating may help. These strategies allow the stomach to completely empty before you lie flat. This may prevent the return of stomach contents into the esophagus, which can cause heartburn. Another commonly given but seldom taken bit of advice is to elevate the head of the bed. This is done by placing bricks or phone books under the head of the bed frame to put the whole bed at a slight angle. I have never met a woman who actually did this, but textbooks say it helps.

Tums or other calcium-containing antacids also work. In the short run, it's fairly hard to overdo these supplements, so chew away. If you find yourself getting constipated, you may need to switch to a different calcium formulation. Everybody responds a little differently, so you can try out various over-the-counter calcium-based antacids until you find one that works for you. Most women (pregnant or not) don't get enough calcium to begin with, so taking these for heartburn will kill two birds with one stone.

Q: *I've tried all those things and nothing seems to help. This acid pain is terrible. I used to take some over-the-counter acid suppressants before I got pregnant. Can I take those now?*

A: Yes, you can. If the strategies mentioned above don't help, it is safe to turn to prescription or over-the-counter acid-suppressant drugs. Researchers examined over 2,000 pregnancies in which women used three common acid suppressors—cimetidine (Tagamet), omeprazole (Prilosec), and ranitidine (Zantac). None of these drugs led to an increase in birth defects. Nor did they increase the chance of preterm delivery or growth problems. In fact, women who took acid suppressors had *fewer* birth defects than other women. So, if Tums or changes in meals don't help, these drugs are worth trying.

Q: *Why does my back hurt so much?*

A: Unfortunately, back pain is very, very common among adults in Western societies. It becomes even more common during pregnancy. Some studies have estimated that one-third of all adults have back pain during their lifetimes. Pregnancy definitely worsens the problem, probably because of the strain on your lower back from the increasing size of the pregnancy. In addition, as your pregnancy progresses, you may become less active or less inclined to move into certain positions. This can cause weakness in the muscles and strain on ligaments, producing pain.

What can you do? Two things will help. First, exercise regularly.

Women who exercise throughout pregnancy have much less back pain. This alone would be a good enough reason to keep exercising throughout pregnancy, but there are other benefits. Women who exercise regularly have easier labors, tend to deliver a few days earlier (and who wouldn't want that?), and have fewer delivery complications. Even a moderate amount of exercise seems to help—you don't need to be training for a marathon.

The second thing that is proved helpful to lessen pain is pain medication (surprise!). Just like when you're not pregnant, taking pain relievers reduces pain. Almost any over-the-counter pain medication can be safely taken for short periods.

Doctors usually recommend Tylenol first, and this is a reasonable place to start. Take enough to help (700 to 1,000 milligrams) and repeat this dose every four hours. If two days of regular dosing has no effect, talk to your doctor about stronger pain medication, usually prescription. Aspirin and ibuprofen should be avoided right around delivery since they can increase bleeding at delivery. If you're more than a couple of weeks away from your due date, aspirin or ibuprofen are fine.

I usually recommend yoga or stretching as treatment for muscular pain as well. The flexibility and muscular strength that come from these activities can reduce pain.

Finally, acupuncture done by a trained acupuncturist appears to be safe in pregnancy and may also be effective in reducing back pain. Dennis Kessler, a Beverly Hills acupuncturist, says, "I've successfully treated many pregnant women for back, neck, and leg pain." He does say that avoiding acupuncture points that stimulate the uterus is easy for any licensed Oriental medical doctor (OMD).

Q: *I have terrible leg cramps, especially at night. What can I do about them?*

A: Despite how many women get these cramps, few good treatments are known. Most treatments involve taking vitamin or mineral supplements under the theory that changes in the body's chemical composition will cause cramps.

Most of the studies of treatments for leg cramps are not randomized trials or don't include a placebo group. Studies that don't include a group treated with placebos don't mean much since many women get better on their own. A study showing that women improve when taking potassium supplements means little unless a similar group of women in the study took a placebo and didn't improve as much. Potassium supplements, for example, haven't been shown to reduce cramps in any well-designed studies. Eating bananas for cramps, a popular folk remedy, hasn't been tested either. But there's no harm in trying.

Nonrandomized studies of calcium treatment also show that these supplements help cramps. However, better designed studies (randomized placebo-controlled trials) of calcium show that it doesn't help. The benefits seen in earlier trials were probably just the placebo effect.

Taking a multivitamin and/or supplement may reduce leg cramps. If you're not taking prenatal vitamins, you might consider starting one. If you already have and you'd like to try magnesium, it is given usually as magnesium lactate or citrate, five to ten milliliters in the morning and evening. Some older studies show that sodium chloride tablets can reduce leg cramps. These days, many women's diets already have so much sodium that I don't recommend taking sodium supplements.

Q: *Constipation is making me miserable. What can I do?*

A: Constipation is a very common problem made worse by routine prescription of prenatal vitamins even when they're not necessary. First, unless you have a specific reason for needing them, stop taking your prenatal vitamins. They can constipate lots of women. And if you have a decent diet, prenatal vitamins don't do you any good after the first trimester (when the folic acid in the vitamins is useful).

If stopping the vitamins doesn't help, all is not lost. Fiber supplements like bran or fiber can reduce constipation and produce softer stools. You mix these products in orange juice or water and drink them. They taste a little bit sandy, but they work. It takes up to a week to see the effect, so don't give up after the first day. An even better way to get more fiber is to eat dates, figs, or prunes.

If adding fiber to your diet and stopping prenatal vitamins doesn't do it, laxatives may help. Unfortunately, the body quickly becomes accustomed to laxatives. If you use them for too long, it can be difficult to move your bowels without them. Severe side effects from laxatives are rare. But I still don't recommend them unless the other approaches don't work.

Q: *My feet are so swollen that I can't even put on my shoes. What should I do?*

A: There are a few things that may combat this common problem. However, because swollen feet can be a sign of preeclampsia (toxemia), check with your doctor to rule out this condition.

The legs and feet swell during pregnancy for a variety of reasons. Some obstetricians say that the feet grow one-half size each pregnancy and never go back. But don't give away your shoes yet. The body takes on extra water during pregnancy and this can cause swelling. The veins change during pregnancy, allowing more fluid to leak out. This fluid accumulates in your feet and legs since they are lower than the rest of your body. These changes will resolve on their own after you deliver.

Some simple strategies can help fight swelling. First, try to cut back on the sodium in your food. Most Americans, pregnant or not, eat too much salt. Most salt comes from prepared foods—not the saltshaker. Fast food usually has way too much sodium. If you eat more than one or two fast food meals a week, you should consider cutting back. The body retains water to compensate for the added sodium and this worsens swelling.

Try to put your feet up above the level of your heart for at least ten minutes four to five times a day. This helps move fluid out of your legs. You may notice that your feet and legs are not as swollen when you first wake up, since the extra fluid gets more evenly distributed while you're lying down.

A more complicated way of getting the same effects uses a device called pneumatic compression stockings. These stockings have multiple air compartments that are inflated and deflated, gradually squeezing the legs and helping to force some of the accumulated fluid out. Wearing these stockings is a big pain so I wouldn't recommend this as a first-line treatment. A simpler method is to soak your whole body in a warm tub.

Water immersion encourages urine production, reducing the amount of fluid retention. Researchers found that fifty minutes of water immersion decreased leg and foot swelling substantially. Adding Epsom salts won't help relieve swelling, but some women like the way it makes the bath feel.

Swimming may help decrease swelling and is great exercise while you're pregnant. If you don't, then this might be the perfect excuse to soak in the tub every night. Tell your husband your doctor ordered it—and he *has* to take care of the kids for a while. Don't be concerned about sitting in the bath for an hour; it's perfectly safe.

Q: *My wrist hurts and some of my fingers are numb. What could be going on?*

A: One of the more common hand ailments that develops during pregnancy is *carpal tunnel syndrome*. The carpal tunnel is a narrow gap between bones in the hand through which runs a major nerve to the hand. Swelling that results from pregnancy can lead to a compression of this nerve through this gap in the bone. When the nerve is sufficiently compressed, you can get pain and numbness in the hand.

It's worth checking this out with your doctor because problems other than carpal tunnel syndrome can cause similar symptoms. Repetitive strain injuries—like those that people who work on assembly lines or as typists get—can also cause hand and wrist pain.

If you do have carpal tunnel syndrome, it's likely to improve after you deliver. Italian researchers studied more than sixty women with proven carpal tunnel syndrome and found that more than half had complete resolution of their symptoms within a year after delivery. The earlier the pregnancy the symptoms started, the less likely they were to resolve after pregnancy.

The first-line treatment for this kind of problem is thorough investigation of causes. In particular, you need to assess whether your hand position during repetitive activities may be contributing to the pain. For example, many typists do not use proper angulation of the wrist and this can lead to hand or wrist problems. It's worth reviewing your daily activities with your doctor, or better yet with a physical therapist to see if any of these activities could be causing the problem. If there's nothing easily identifiable that can be modified to reduce your pain, then over-the-counter pain relievers are a good first-line treatment. If these fail, then wrist splinting is also worth a try. Occupational therapists at the Darnall Army Community Hospital in Fort Hood, Texas found that splinting helped reduce pain and increase grip strength in women with carpal tunnel syndrome during pregnancy. Surgery is rarely recommended during pregnancy for carpal tunnel syndrome unless the problem predated the pregnancy. In many cases, the problem will resolve after delivery, so performing surgery should be a last resort.

In short, hand and wrist problems may be common during pregnancy and the best solution usually involves identifying causal factors and trying to change those. Physical therapists and occupational therapists are probably the most useful practitioners to seek help from about this condition. If your problem started during pregnancy, the odds are good it will disappear after you deliver.

Q: *I'm having a huge amount of pain right over my pubic bone. Is that from the baby's head pushing against it?*

A: It's hard to know exactly the cause of this kind of pain, but it is fairly common during pregnancy. The hormone *relaxin* helps loosen the pelvic joints and allows the pelvis to widen slightly during delivery. Some people think midline pubic pain come from the resultant softening or loosening of the joint between the two pubic bones.

The pain will go away. A Danish study of more than 1,700 pregnant women found that all of the women with midline pain over the pubic bone felt better within six months of delivery. In the meantime, taking over-the-counter pain medication may help. Some physical therapists and midwives suggest pelvic tilting exercises to help strengthen the pelvic ligaments during pregnancy. These exercises may also help relieve pain over the pubic bone. Look for a physical therapist who treats pregnant women to get help with these types of exercises.

Q: *Why do I have so much vaginal discharge? I'm afraid I might have an infection.*

A: You might have an infection, and it's worth checking this out with your prenatal care provider. You may also be experiencing a change in the amount and type of vaginal discharge that is perfectly normal for pregnancy.

Most women, pregnant or not, experience some type of vaginal discharge. The discharge contains mostly dead skin cells from the vagina and from the cervix. During pregnancy, the amount of discharge increases. More skin cells sloughing off and more cervical mucus explain this increase.

Women get more candida, or yeast infections, during pregnancy. These infections are easily treated if the discharge is bothersome. Yeast poses no risk to you or your baby, so if the discharge is not bothersome, treatment may not be necessary. Vaginal yeast infections do not cause oral yeast infections, or thrush, in either baby or mother.

Bacterial vaginosis can also increase or change the vaginal discharge. Bacterial vaginosis, like candida, can be safely treated during pregnancy. If you've had a previous preterm delivery and have bacterial vaginosis, then getting treated may reduce your risk of another preterm delivery. The antibiotic used to treat bacterial vaginosis is safe in pregnancy.

Sexually transmitted diseases like gonorrhea and chlamydia can also increase vaginal discharge. These infections absolutely must be treated if detected, otherwise the baby can be infected during delivery.

Most of the time, a change in vaginal discharge is simply a normal part of pregnancy. Nonetheless, you should bring these changes to your provider's attention so he or she can rule out any treatable infections.

Q: *I want to have sex all the time but I'm seven months pregnant. Is this safe? Am I normal?*

A: Yes on both counts. Both men and women may experience an increase in sexual desire through the course of pregnancy. For many couples, it's the first time they don't need to worry about birth control. Lack of communication can sometimes get in the way of acting on sexual urges. A woman who feels overweight or out of shape may not realize that her partner finds her *more* desirable. Some men wonder if it's safe to act on their sexual urges, or have been warned that sex will hurt the baby.

The developing fetus is well protected inside the uterus. Except under very specific circumstances, sexual intercourse is safe during pregnancy. Doctors used to say that having sex could begin labor—but it's not nearly that simple! Many couples try to bring on labor with sex but it doesn't work very well. Sex does increase uterine contractions but these contractions just slow down and fade away.

You shouldn't have sexual intercourse if you are having unexplained vaginal bleeding or have ruptured membranes. In either of these cases, you should talk to your doctor immediately—having sex is the least of your worries. If you have placenta previa, a condition where the placenta covers the opening of the cervix, then you should discuss with your doctor whether sex is safe or not. Some doctors also recommend not having sex if you've been treated for preterm labor. But sex does not cause labor and there is no evidence to substantiate this advice. Unless your cervix is dilated to more than three centimeters and you are more than six weeks away from delivery, having sex is still safe.

Unless your doctor specifically tells you not to, you should be able to continue having sex throughout pregnancy.

Q: *My husband and I tried to get pregnant for two years. When we finally did, it seems like we just stopped having sex. Do you think things will get back to normal?*

A: Absolutely. What you're describing is very common. Many of my patients who had a hard time getting pregnant were so relieved when they did that they just stopped making love. I think they had started to think of having sex as very "goal driven." Once they reached their goal, they just stopped. Research confirms this. A study showed that couples who spent a long time trying to conceive had sex less during pregnancy.

Things will get back to normal. Between six and twelve months after delivery, most couples are having sex at about the same frequency as they did before pregnancy.

Q: *I'm five months pregnant and I'm not even showing. What's wrong with me?*

A: Keep your voice down. Many women would kill to be in your situation. As long as you have been going to your doctor regularly and he or she has confirmed that your pregnancy is progressing normally, you have nothing to worry about. Pregnancy affects each woman's body differently. Some women tend to gain weight early in their pregnancy, others seem to gain it later. The uterus may be in a slightly different position in different women. This too can affect how "pregnant" you look.

At five months, your fetus, placenta, and amniotic fluid probably weigh one pound altogether. So in some sense, it is remarkable that it is *ever* possible to tell that a woman is pregnant at this stage. The bottom line: *don't worry*. Your doctor probably measures your uterus at every visit and will tell you if he or she sees a problem. Just be happy that you haven't had to shell out for new clothes yet.

Q: *Does vitamin E work to get rid of stretch marks?*

A: Probably not. Nobody has yet found an effective way to get rid of "stretch marks" that often accompany pregnancy.

Interestingly, stretch marks are not simply a result of stretching. They do tend to appear where the skin has been distended or stretched rapidly, like in pregnancy or in people with rapid weight gain. But they also seem to be related to hormone changes. The often purplish color that accompanies pregnancy stretch marks may be a result of high hormone levels during pregnancy.

Looked at under a microscope, these marks look like tiny scars. Almost every treatment that has been used to try to prevent scarring after surgery has been used to try to prevent stretch marks during pregnancy. None of them works very well. The good news is that stretch marks fade after pregnancy. Within a year, they are hardly noticeable. If discoloration remains, then intense pulsed laser therapy (which can be given by a dermatologist) can improve the appearance of these marks.

Vitamin E, cocoa butter, Vaseline, or any other topical therapies don't help much. On the other hand, they won't hurt, and if they make you feel better, go ahead and use them.

Q: *Why do I have to pee all the time?*

A: Your need to urinate, assuming you don't have a bladder infection, is affected by three main things. First, how much fluid you're taking in—if you drink the eight glasses of water a day that some people recommend, I'm not surprised you have to pee constantly. Second, the ability of your bladder to expand to hold urine—and your expanding uterus reduces the space available for the bladder. Third, the nerve impulses that your bladder sends to and receives from your brain.

Drinking large amounts of fluid contributes to urinary frequency. Read the section on water consumption in Chapter Six for a more detailed discussion, but you should drink enough not to feel thirsty. Don't feel compelled to drink an arbitrary amount of water (like eight 8-ounce glasses a day). Drinking this much won't help your pregnancy a bit.

Compression of the bladder by an enlarging uterus commonly makes women pee more frequently. As the uterus grows, it presses on all the neighboring organs. The empty bladder acts like a deflated balloon and doesn't take up much space. As it expands with urine, it needs a place to go. By the third trimester of pregnancy, this area has gotten much tighter (see illustration). There's not much you can do about this.

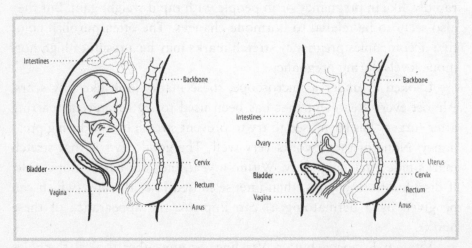

Figure 6

Changes in nerve function during pregnancy can also lead to urinary frequency. Normally, when the bladder expands to a certain point, the stretching muscle fibers cause nerve impulses to be sent to your brain, telling you it's time to empty your bladder. Most people don't get an overwhelming urge to urinate until the bladder is filled with a cup and a half to two cups of urine. During pregnancy, these nerve impulses might begin sooner, leading to an urge to urinate at a cup or so. Trying to wait a little bit longer each time before you urinate may quiet these impulses.

But don't wait too long—or a pregnancy-related decrease in your bladder control might come into play!

Q: *Why do I pee every time I cough or laugh?*

A: One of the many things that pregnancy can do is reduce your ability to control your urine. "Continence," or the ability to hold your urine, comes from a combination of muscles and nerves in the bladder working together in a coordinated way. It appears that pregnancy affects both the muscles *and* the nerves, making it harder to "stay dry" in certain circumstances. Coughing and laughing both increase the pressure on your bladder. Normally, when this pressure increases, your bladder muscles can keep things under control. When you're pregnant, this increase in pressure overwhelms your body's ability to hold your urine.

Most women experience this unpleasant change in the way the body works during pregnancy. Researchers at the University of North Carolina in Chapel Hill studied 123 women throughout pregnancy. In the first trimester, about one in ten women leaked when coughing; by the third trimester more than half did. By eight weeks after delivery, the number was down to one in five. (Other studies have shown that it takes up to six months for normal bladder function to return after delivery, so some of the women who were still leaking at eight weeks probably improved later, but this particular study didn't measure it.)

Many doctors recommend Kegel exercises to reduce these symptoms. Kegels are done by tightening and loosening the muscles that control the stream of urine. Unfortunately, Kegels done during pregnancy don't

Dealing With Your Changing Body

- Backaches, headaches, and other pains can be safely treated with ibuprofen (Advil or Motrin), aspirin, or acetominophen (Tylenol)
- For heartburn, try Tums or other antacids. If these don't work, consider over-the-counter acid suppressors, like omeprazole.
- Constipation may improve if you stop your prenatal vitamins and increase your fiber intake (ideally in foods, but fiber supplements work too)
- Cutting down on salt and soaking in the tub can reduce leg and foot swelling.
- Unless your doctor specifically tells you not to, you can continue to have sex throughout pregnancy. Sex does not cause labor—preterm or at term.

do much to control urine leakage. For whatever reason, these muscular exercises can't overcome the changes associated with pregnancy.

If you are still having problems after delivery, Kegels should help, but starting them while you're still pregnant doesn't seem to do anything. It may be that the changes in bladder function during pregnancy are too great to be overcome by these exercises, or that changes in nerves rather than muscles are mostly responsible. Kegel exercises may strengthen the right muscles, but if the nerves aren't playing along, you may still leak.

Involuntary urine loss during pregnancy may be embarrassing, but it's very common and there doesn't appear to be much that improves it. You may be able to "work around it" by emptying your bladder sooner than you usually would. This reduces the amount of urine your bladder has to hold and may reduce the frequency of urine loss. Mostly though, you'll have to wait until after delivery to see an improvement.

11 You Can't Get There From Here:

Getting Around Town
(or Out of Town) Safely

"It is better to travel well than to arrive."—Buddha

Traveling while pregnant brings with it a whole series of potential problems. Travel has become part of the fabric of our everyday lives to such an extent that these questions have become more and more common. Countless pregnant women have faced the issue of deciding when it's "too late" to travel. Airlines may have one answer, your doctor another, and your best friend a third. This chapter explains the issues underlying concerns about travel in pregnancy. It examines each potential problem that can result and helps you think through what makes sense for you. The answers in this chapter will let you make sense of the conflicting advice you get on this very common topic.

Q: *I was told I shouldn't wear my seat belt when my belly gets big because in an accident, it might hurt my baby.*

A: You sure didn't hear that from me. The most common cause of fetal death is maternal death and about two to three percent of pregnant women are involved in motor vehicle accidents during the course of their pregnancies, making car crashes one of the most dangerous things in pregnancy. Car crashes are far more dangerous to a pregnant women than any medication you could accidentally take during pregnancy, drinking coffee, changing your cat litter, or almost any other potentially or supposedly risky activity that we've covered in this book. In other words, the most important way to keep your baby alive and well is for *you* to stay alive and well.

Wearing a seat belt is an absolute must—pregnant or not. The lap belt should go below your belly and the shoulder belt above. (See illustration.) But how you wear your belt doesn't matter nearly as much as *whether* you wear it. Your baby is very well protected inside your uterus. It is very rare for a fetus to be injured in an accident that doesn't injure the mother. That's another way of saying that if you stay safe, your baby stays safe.

Air bags and seat belts save mothers and babies. Researchers at the University of Michigan extensively studied car crashes involving pregnant women. They confirmed that the worse the crash, the more likely the fetus is to be injured. They also found that being belted and/or having an air bag dramatically improved the chances that both mother and baby come out OK. The vast majority of car crashes occur at speeds of less than fifteen miles an hour (minor) or fifteen to thirty miles an hour (moderate). In these crashes, proper use of air bags and seat belts dramatically reduces fetal injury. In one study, in moderate crashes with an unrestrained mother, nearly all of the fetuses were injured. On the other hand, if the mother was restrained, about seventy percent of the fetuses

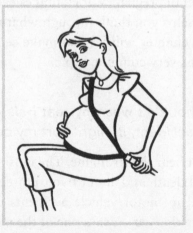

Figure 7

had no injury. In minor crashes, the injury rate was fifty percent for the fetus if the mother wasn't restrained and only ten percent if she was. In severe crashes, air bags and seat belts may not matter, because these crashes often severely injure or kill the mother regardless of restraint.

Q: *What about air bags? Can an expanding air bag hurt my baby?*

A: Air bags are a major safety innovation. They reduce the risk of death in accidents. They were originally designed to reduce injury to an unbelted passenger about the size of an average man. Because of this design, they may cause injury (or even death) in very rare situations. Being pregnant is *not* one of these situations.

Air bags were originally designed for the average person in an average accident. That is, they are supposed to protect an unseatbelted adult in a high-speed frontal collision. Children and smaller adults (less than 100 pounds) can be hurt if they are struck by the expanding air bag. Automobile companies make "smarter" air bags these days—reducing or eliminating this risk. But even riding in a car with a "first generation" air bag is safer than being in a car without them. Slamming your belly against the dashboard or steering wheel is worse than slamming into an air bag.

There are some rare situations where an air bag could hurt you. For example, if you are in a low-speed crash and are not wearing your seat belt, the force of the air bag could be greater than the force you would have experienced hitting the dash. Avoiding air bags to avoid this rare situation is like not wearing your seat belt so you can "be thrown clear of the car" in a crash—both are stupid ideas. Air bags help hundreds or thousands of times as many people as they hurt. A smarter thing to do (pregnant or not) would be to wear your seat belt and push the seat back as far as possible from the dashboard.

Q: *Can I travel in an airplane during pregnancy?*

A: Absolutely. Air travel presents no measurable risk to your developing fetus. But you may want to limit travel toward the end of your pregnancy for two reasons. First, you'll probably want to be close to home. Second, sitting for long periods can increase your risk of developing blood clots in your legs. (But sitting while driving has the same effect, so if you're traveling long distances, flying is safer.)

According to a recent study in the journal *Obstetrics & Gynecology*, fewer than one in 1,000 pregnant women develops a blood clot in their legs during pregnancy. Even if prolonged air travel doubles this risk, that's still only two women in 1,000. If you do fly, you can probably lower your risk to one in 1,000 with a few simple precautions. First get up and move around frequently in flight (often easier to do in the air than on a long drive). Second, point and flex your toes every few minutes (this tenses and relaxes the calf muscles, which are responsible for keeping blood from pooling in your legs where it may clot).

The most dangerous consequence of getting a blood clot in the leg is that the clot can travel to your lungs. This problem (called "pulmonary embolism") occurs most commonly in the two months *after* you've delivered. So waiting until after the baby is born to take your trip is worse than going late in pregnancy. Overall, the odds are about 10,000 to one against you getting blood clots in your lungs, whether you fly or not.

Q: *What is "coach class syndrome" and does it affect me?*

A: "Coach class syndrome" is the sound-bite term for the blood clots in the legs mentioned above. A recent study linked these blood clots and long flights in coach for certain groups of people (like people over fifty or those with certain medical problems). It does apply to pregnancy in a way (although the researchers who invented that term didn't study pregnant women), because the blood does clot more easily during pregnancy. When you walk, blood is pumped back to your heart by the squeezing action of your leg muscles. Staying still in a plane seat means you're not using your leg muscles much and blood can stay longer in your legs than usual. If the blood stays too long, a clot can develop. "Coach class" doesn't really have much to do with it. Moving to first class might get you better food, but it won't reduce your risk of clots.

Recommendations for Safe Airline Travel in Pregnancy

From the Royal College of Obstetricians and Gynecologists

Short Haul
(Flights less than or equal to three hours)
Calf exercises
Move around frequently
Avoid dehydration

Long Haul
(Flights greater than four hours)
Calf exercises
Move around frequently
Avoid dehydration
Wear elastic below-knee compression stockings

Women with Additional Risk Factors*

All of the above plus wear elastic below-knee compression stockings

All of the above plus consider Heparin (a blood thinner) on the day of and the day after travel.

*Additional risk factors include: Weight greater than 220 pound. • Twins or other multiple pregnancy • Medical problems that lead to increased risk of blood clotting (discuss with your doctor) • Blood-clotting problems • Strong family history of blood-clotting problems.

You can reduce your risk without upgrading. Get up and move around every fifteen minutes or so (get an aisle seat if you can). Ask for bulkhead seating where there is more legroom (these seats are sometimes held for people with disabilities). And make a habit of pointing and flexing your toes every few minutes while you're sitting. These things pump the blood through your legs and will probably prevent any problems.

Q: *Doesn't flying increase the risk of preterm labor?*

A: The closer to your due date you are, the more likely you'll go into labor while traveling. But flying itself has no effect on when labor starts. Decisions about travel during pregnancy require more common sense than medical knowledge. A two-hour plane flight on your due date to a city where you have identified a doctor in advance is no more dangerous than living in a rural area with the closest hospital two hours away. It may be less dangerous, depending on how your husband drives.

Of course, many airlines (and many doctors) still say you shouldn't travel after thirty-six weeks of pregnancy. I think you should do what you want, as long as it's safe. And air travel is as safe as it gets.

The airlines, of course, have one good reason for not wanting you onboard after thirty-six weeks—namely, they don't want to turn a Boeing 747 into a flying labor and delivery ward. Neither do you, because even if you're lucky enough to be flying with an obstetrician—the odds are against you getting an epidural at 30,000 feet.

Q: *A stewardess told me I shouldn't fly because of the "radiation" exposure. What is she talking about?*

A: Flying exposes you to small amounts of radiation, but not enough to worry about. The radiation comes from outer space, believe it or not. Cosmic rays continually pepper us with radiation, but the atmosphere absorbs most of it. When you're 30,000 feet up in the air, there's less atmosphere around, so more radiation gets to you. A woman living in Denver gets more radiation than one living in New York, and someone flying in a plane gets more than someone on the ground.

Is it risky? No. One study found a slight increase in miscarriage risk in women (usually flight attendants) who flew seventy-five hours or more per *month*. The risk identified in this study was of miscarriage in the first ten weeks of pregnancy. In other words, any risk is highest in early pregnancy—not what most people would guess—and only very frequent flyers have an increased risk.

The Federal Aviation Authority (FAA) suggests that pregnant women limit this radiation exposure to one-tenth of the maximum allowed when not pregnant. You would have to fly 75,000 miles during your pregnancy to reach this limit. As a result, for most travelers flying presents no significant radiation risk to a fetus.

Safe Traveling While Pregnant

- Seat belts save lives—never drive without one.
- Use your shoulder belt, it won't hurt your baby in a crash and it could save your life.
- Air bag–equipped seats are safer than seats without air bags.
- With few exceptions, it's safe to fly during pregnancy, and mile for mile, airplanes are by far the safest way to travel.

If you have already logged quite a few miles and are concerned, consider this: The FAA calculates that even hitting that 75,000-mile maximum only increases the risk of fetal problems by three in 10,000. Putting this into context, in the general population more than 300 out of 10,000 babies have major or minor abnormalities at birth. In other words, even flying the maximum recommended number of miles during your pregnancy increases your overall risk by less than one percent.

Q: *Are there any circumstances in which I shouldn't fly?*

A: Yes, but they are rare. Flying on long commercial flights at high altitudes results in a slightly lower oxygen delivery to the fetus. You needn't be concerned about this lower oxygen level except under some specific circumstances. Fetal blood very effectively traps and stores oxygen, allowing it to handle short periods of lower oxygen levels easily.

However, if there are placental or fetal abnormalities that already lower the fetus's oxygen supply, then even short periods of air travel could be hazardous. These abnormalities are rare and should be identifiable by your doctor. Specifically, growth retardation, evidence of fetal distress, preeclampsia, or poorly treated diabetes all may indicate lower oxygen delivery. In these circumstances, the reduced oxygen the fetus faces during airplane travel might become significant.

If travel is medically necessary or urgent, then a commercial flight is safer than traveling the same distance by car. If you have one of the problems listed above, then your doctor can prescribe supplemental oxygen. If worn throughout the flight, this will more than compensate for reduced oxygen at high altitudes.

Q: *How late in pregnancy is too late to travel?*

A: It depends. If your pregnancy is progressing normally and you feel well, then it's really never too late. The main question to ask yourself is, "How comfortable do I feel having my baby wherever I'm going?" If you feel fine with it, it's probably okay to go.

Many obstetricians pick arbitrary limits (like thirty-six weeks) after which they suggest their patients not travel. It's fine to adhere to these limits, but most women are capable of understanding that this is just a common sense number—not a scientific statement of safety. If you want to visit a major city with a big hospital at thirty-seven weeks, what could the danger be? If you don't want to deliver your baby in another city, then sure, don't go. But don't cancel your plans just because you've passed some arbitrary date.

On the other hand, many women don't want to leave the bedroom after a certain point in pregnancy, much less travel to another city. This "nesting" feeling is very normal. Combine nesting with the fatigue you're likely to have at the end of pregnancy, and wanting to stay put is quite understandable. Despite the "safety" of traveling, you should still feel comfortable declining to go somewhere or do something because of your pregnancy. This is an important time and you should follow your instincts. If you don't want to go someplace, you can always say your doctor recommended that you not go. Almost everyone will give you extra leeway when you're pregnant; don't hesitate to use it!

When Traveling Abroad

- Try to identify a doctor in your destination city before you go.
- Copy your prenatal record and bring it with you.
- Bring your regular doctor's phone number with you.
- Remember that pregnancy outcomes are *better* in many European countries than in the United States.

Q: *I'm pregnant with twins. What travel precautions should I take?*

A: Being pregnant with twins puts you at higher risk for a variety of problems, like growth retardation (meaning slower than normal growth of one or both fetuses) and preterm labor. While there still aren't hard and fast rules about what you can and can't do, in general, you should be more cautious than someone with a singleton pregnancy.

If your obstetrician has been following you closely and hasn't found any problems, then traveling in the second trimester (up to twenty-four weeks) is probably safe enough. After that, it's anyone's guess. Most obstetricians who deal with twin pregnancies have developed their own sense of what they do or don't feel comfortable with and you should use this as your guide. Don't be afraid to ask your doctor why he or she doesn't want you to do something. Sometimes, just explaining why you want to go will initiate a discussion about why your doctor doesn't feel it's safe.

Q: *What about other pregnancy complications? How do these affect when I should stay close to home?*

A: If you have certain complications of pregnancy, like preterm labor, ruptured membranes, or some condition that requires frequent monitoring of your baby, I'd say that it's already too late. Any time you interrupt your medical treatment, or put many miles between you and your doctor, you make it much more difficult to respond quickly to new developments. This is the time for you to stick close to home. If you desperately need a getaway, make it local: One night in a hotel or bed-and-breakfast not far from home can sometimes do wonders for the psyche.

Q: *I'm supposed to be in a wedding in Spain when I'm eight months pregnant. Should I go?*

A: The answer to this question depends on so many different factors, like how important it is to you that your mother not think you're crazy, and how close you are to the person getting married.

Most doctors would simply tell you that you shouldn't go. If your doctor says this, ask her why. I think her reason could be summed up like this: "Well, what if something happens?" To which I would respond: "Something like what?"

Let's think about what you're facing with a trip to Europe. First, a long plane flight. Flying isn't inherently dangerous, and with some simple precautions it can be done pretty much throughout pregnancy. But if the thought of flying that distance puts you off, you need not read on. Just tell your friend that your doctor says you can't go. What true friend would argue with that?

If you're not afraid to fly, let's see what's next. Once you land, you'll be in an unfamiliar country where you may not speak the language, and where you may go into labor.

Rest assured that women in Spain have babies all the time without any apparent ill effects. (Spain—along with Sweden, Ireland, and a variety of other European countries—has *lower* maternal and infant mortality rates than the United States.) The signs of labor are unmistakable in any language.

Knowledge is power. The best way to handle foreign travel is to prepare. Before you leave, contact the American Embassy in the country you're visiting (you can get their number from the State Department—see the **Resources** section). Find out if there are any obstetricians they recommend, or that had their training in America. Copy your medical record and bring it with you. Most of all, remember that the maternal and fetal death or injury rates are lower in some other countries than they are here. You'll be in unfamiliar territory, it's true. But think of the stories you'll tell your baby when he or she is old enough!

1 2 Work, Work, Work:

Making It Through the Workday

"The brain is a wonderful organ; it starts working the moment you get up in the morning and does not stop until you get into the office."—Robert Frost

For decades the number of women working outside the home has been increasing. More women in the workforce means more pregnant women in the workplace. Concerns about working during pregnancy usually depend on the type of work being done. Some women sit at computers all day and wonder if there is radiation coming from the screen. Women whose work involves lifting or physical activity often wonder when, or if, these activities can become dangerous. Almost every woman, working or not, deals with an extra helping of fatigue during pregnancy. Managing this fatigue can be particularly hard for working women. This chapter gives the answers that women who work outside the home need in order to make it safely through pregnancy.

Q: *How can I explain to my boss that even though I'm only ten weeks pregnant, by 3 o'clock I'm so tired I can't function at work anymore?*

A: This is an all-too-common problem. Over the last generation, there has been an explosion of women who get and stay pregnant while continuing to work. To date, researchers have done far too few studies on the effects of working throughout pregnancy. Two existing studies that examined the effect of work on pregnancy found (not surprisingly) a link between working and increased fatigue.

Ninety-seven percent of pregnant women report being fatigued in the first trimester, eighty-nine percent in the second trimester, eighty-seven percent in the third trimester, and eighty-eight percent after delivery. Almost everyone is fatigued throughout their entire pregnancy. I'm not suggesting that you should just "suck it up," but rather that you have plenty of company.

Before you accept your fatigue as a natural part of your pregnancy, make sure you don't have any conditions that could make you more tired. Anemia and lack of sleep are the most common culprits here. A blood count will pick up anemia and iron supplements will usually fix it. Most obstetricians check for anemia once or twice in the course of pregnancy.

Lack of sleep is harder to fix. If you're having trouble sleeping, you should get into bed only when you're tired and get out if you can't sleep. Make sure it's dark in your bedroom. Wear a blackout mask if you can't control the lighting. Some sleeping aids (like Benadryl and Unisom) are safe during pregnancy. If you don't sleep enough because you "don't have time," then the fix is even easier: make time. Most people need eight hours of sleep a night—many pregnant women need an hour more. There are no short cuts—you have to go to bed earlier. Cut out television. You'll feel better with an hour more sleep and an hour less tube.

Unfortunately, fatigue is a normal part of pregnancy, and may be the body's way of telling you to get extra rest. If you're lucky, your boss will be understanding and give you opportunities to take breaks. If not, you'll have to make them on your own.

Q: *I'm a lawyer in a busy law firm, and I've already had one miscarriage. Should I stop working in order to improve my chances of staying pregnant?*

A: Professional women like you are in a difficult situation. Many such women feel internal and external pressure to continue working even when they shouldn't. Wage-earning employees can often take time off work with a note from their doctor. Doctors and lawyers find it almost impossible to do this.

Surprisingly little research has been done on the effect work has on pregnancy, despite how many women now work outside the home. Most of these studies are of poor quality and therefore difficult to interpret. In general, studies show that extremes of physical activity, including heavy lifting (carrying loads of over twenty pounds), lifting items more than fifteen times a day, standing for more than eight hours a day (like when working a shift on an assembly line), and other types of heavy physical effort slightly increase the risk of spontaneous abortion.

Better studies must be done to confirm that these activities are truly risky. Nonetheless, if your position requires these activities and you are trying to get pregnant, try to switch to one that does not. (Many employers will make temporary changes if given a doctor's note.) Some studies show that night work increases the risk of miscarriage, so you should consider requesting day shifts until you deliver.

This advice doesn't help the lawyer who works a stressful job but does not do any heavy lifting. Although we all understand the term "stress," it is difficult to measure precisely. Because it can't be easily measured, researchers have a hard time studying it. Studies of the effect of this kind of stress in pregnancy just don't exist.

I firmly believe that reducing job stress can only help your chances of keeping a pregnancy. Discuss your concerns with your doctor and ask her to write a letter explaining that your pregnancy outcome might depend on reducing your hours and/or stress level. Your partners may not be happy with your decision to cut back, but I think it's a good decision. With the doctor's note, your partners will probably be supportive.

Q: *I've heard that working with computers can be dangerous because of the radiation. What should I do to protect myself?*

A: In the 1980s, there were reports of a variety of bad pregnancy outcomes linked to computer and video screens. Since that time, more data have been collected that disproves those early reports. Using computers or electronic terminals poses no risk to your pregnancy.

Early reports identified four main concerns: increased risk of abortion, lower birth weight, increased risk of preterm delivery, and increased birth defects. The best current evidence is that the use of computers or video units does not cause any of these adverse outcomes. Researchers recently examined all of the studies on this topic (studies that included more than 30,000 women) and found no increased risk at all. So, you can surf the Internet for fascinating facts about pregnancy and feel perfectly safe doing it!

Q: *I'm required to fly for my job (more than 100,000 miles a year). Is it dangerous to fly this much?*

A: Other than crashing (the risk of which is extremely small), the greatest danger from air travel is exposure to solar radiation. During the very early part of pregnancy (the first eight weeks), the fetus is particularly susceptible to radiation exposure. It's very hard to measure, but your travel might increase your risk from this exposure—but the increase is tiny. The FAA recommends a maximum radiation dose for airline crews, and this limit is not reached unless the crew member flies more than 300,000 miles in a year.

At 100,000 miles per year, your travel may present a very small increase in your risk and your fetus's risk of some adverse outcomes. Theoretically, your travel might increase your lifetime risk of cancer by about one percent. The risk of birth defects in your fetus might be similarly elevated. Not a one percent chance that you or your baby will have problems, but a one percent *greater* chance than if you didn't fly. Three out of 100,000 babies are born with some birth defect. A one percent increase means 303 (instead of 300) in every 100,000 babies having a birth defect.

I wish I could provide a simpler answer. The bottom line is that extensive travel presents some risk, but that the risk is very small.

Q: *I'm a dentist and we use mercury in the office. Is this exposure dangerous to my pregnancy?*

A: Mercury toxicity can affect the fetal nervous system, so you are right to be concerned. The Occupational Safety and Health Administration (OSHA) sets limits on mercury in the workplace to protect people like you. Most people's main mercury exposure comes from food (fish in particular). The FDA has recently set recommended limits on the amount of fish that pregnant women should eat.

Workplace mercury exposure can lead to toxicity, so overexposure from workplace sources is possible. OSHA sets the same limits for pregnant and nonpregnant women, but pregnant women might want to be extra cautious.

If you work with mercury, have your blood or urine tested for mercury levels. Most women in the general population have blood mercury levels of less than two micrograms per deciliter and urine levels of less than ten micrograms per deciliter. If your levels are higher than this, consider staying away from mercury (by limiting your workplace exposure and your fish consumption).

Q: *I used to do quite a bit of painting and was thinking of taking it up again, but I'm worried about the effect it might have on my pregnancy. Is exposure to paint and paint thinner dangerous?*

A: It's not dangerous to paint your house, have it professionally painted, or visit somebody else whose house is being painted. On the other hand, being a professional painter does appear to have some risk.

Studies of organic solvents (commonly used in paint thinners) suggest that they can increase the risk of malformations in a developing fetus. In fact, women who had consistent and regular exposure to organic solvents had *thirteen times* the risk of major birth defects compared with women without exposure.

I would discourage pregnant women (or women trying to get pregnant) from working in places where organic solvents are used. Many factory workers, lab technicians, artists, painters, and chemists have such exposure. Federal law requires employers to tell workers about their exposure. If you think organic solvents are in use in your workplace, request a list of the chemicals used from your employer. Discuss the list with your doctor, or contact a national or regional poison control center (see **Resources**) to help decide if you're at risk.

Q: *My work is physically demanding and includes lifting boxes and climbing ladders. How can I stay safe?*

A: Physically demanding work can increase your risk of miscarriage, so don't wait until late in pregnancy to try to change your job responsibilities. Women who work at physically demanding jobs during pregnancy may be more likely to be injured on the job. Pregnancy can strain the lower back. Fluid retention and hand swelling can contribute to carpal tunnel syndrome.

Heavy lifting may increase the risk of miscarriages and preterm delivery. It may increase the risk of growth retardation and high blood pressure. Thirty percent more women who work in physically demanding jobs will have these complications than women who don't work in such jobs. Not a huge increase, but big enough that you should try to reduce or avoid such work.

Talk with your doctor. Ask for a note stating that your workload may endanger your pregnancy. It's the rare employer who won't take a doctor's note from a pregnant woman seriously. They should accommodate you and help you find another job or role that doesn't require these activities.

Pregnancy is not an illness, but it can increase your susceptibility to certain problems. Reducing work stress, especially physical stress, can help improve the chance of a good outcome.

Q: *Some people say exercise is good for you in pregnancy but you're saying that physically demanding work should be limited. What's the story?*

A: Voluntary physical activity (like exercise) improves your heart health but working in a physically demanding job doesn't. Similarly, during pregnancy, recreational physical activity and work-related activity have different effects on your body.

Exercise is fundamentally different from work. Exercise decreases stress, but work-related activity usually increases it. In addition, most recreational activity doesn't result in severe fatigue, whereas excessive work activity can. Finally, most people work for more hours than they exercise.

Women who exercise during pregnancy have fewer complaints about aches and pains, less fatigue, shorter labors, and fewer labor complications. Women with physically demanding jobs, on the other hand, have a slightly higher miscarriage rate and may have higher rates of preterm delivery. Exercise makes you feel good: Common sense would tell you that is probably a good thing. Work-related activity often makes you feel exhausted, so this may not be quite as good of a thing.

Q: *I drive for several hours a day as part of my job. Should I try to get a desk job while I'm pregnant?*

A: I don't think so. I've never seen any studies linking driving with pregnancy complications. However, pregnant women have a higher risk of blood clots forming in the legs. Being confined in a small space without much movement for an extended period causes blood to pool in the veins in your legs. This pooled blood can form clots, blocking off some of the veins. The actual chance of this happening is very, very small but is higher in people who are immobile for long periods of time. (For example, by flying on long flights, or by being immobilized by a broken leg.)

Moving the feet up and down at the ankles, like when you press on the gas and brake, contracts and relaxes the muscles in the calf, helping to pump blood out of the legs and back toward the heart. When you drive, you're doing this work all the time. Unless you crash your car—which should be no more likely now that you're pregnant—you're probably safe with your current job.

Q: *I work in a restaurant. Are there foods I should avoid preparing? I've heard that handling certain foods could infect my baby.*

A: If you follow the usual food preparation guidelines (washing your hands frequently with soap and hot water, not sampling foods as you prepare them), you will be fine. There are very few infections that can actually pass from the mother to the fetus. Only one of these infections typically comes from food—*Listeria monocytogenes,* which can cause miscarriage in early pregnancy. Listeria sometimes contaminates soft cheeses, unpasteurized milk products, and some deli meats. Preparation of these foods, however, *does not* put you at risk for Listeria infection. Eating them does. Listeria infection is very rare (fewer than 100 Listeria infections occurred in the United States last year), but if you avoid eating the foods noted, your risk will be just about zero.

Q: *I work with plastics a lot. Can this could be dangerous for the baby?*

A: No. Plastics pose no significant health risk.

A U.S. government agency called the Center for Evaluation of Risks to Human Reproduction recently completed a study on the effect of certain plastic byproducts. Called phthalates, these byproducts come from chemicals used to make plastic softer and more flexible. Phthalates can leak into water or fluids stored in plastic containers. Phthalates used to package foods also make their way into the body. You may have heard people saying that you shouldn't use plastic containers to heat foods in the microwave. Phthalates are the reason for these statements.

Plastics are everywhere in our society. While more studies are needed, there is no evidence that they can hurt pregnant women. The government panel that reviewed the risks concluded that plastic byproducts *may* be hazardous but that no good studies have been done. In animal studies, large doses of these chemicals caused birth defects.

If there is a risk, it's a small one. I wouldn't recommend changing your habits because of concerns over the toxic effects of plastics. When you eliminate something, you have to replace it with something else. If you don't use plastics, you might increase your use of glass products. If phthalates from plastics harm one out of every 100,000 people who use them, and glass causes severe cuts in one out of 10,000 people, then plastic might really be safer!

This example may sound silly, but it illustrates the dilemma that we face when examining a risk without examining the alternatives. Good

Resources for Women With
Workplace Chemical Exposure

Organization	Website	Phone Number
Motherisk	www.motherisk.org	(416) 813-6780
Organization of Teratology Information Services	www.OTISpregnancy.org	(888) 285-3410
Occupational Health and Safety Administration	www.osha.gov	(800) 321-OSHA

scientific studies will always try to include the risk of some alternative when identifying the exposure risk.

While the subject deserves more study, plastics belong near the bottom of the list of things to worry about during pregnancy.

Q: *Is it dangerous to work in a hair salon if I'm trying to get pregnant?*

A: It doesn't appear to be. A fifteen-year-old study showed an increased risk of miscarriage in some women who worked as cosmetologists. Women who worked more than forty hours a week, stood for more than eight hours a day, or did a large number of hair treatments had a slightly higher risk of miscarriage than did other women. More recent studies have not found the same thing. Changes in dye formulas and rules requiring better ventilation may have made hairdressers safer, or the earlier studies may have been mistaken.

Just to be safe, take some simple precautions. Wear gloves when using chemical treatments. Make sure that your room is well ventilated. Take frequent breaks so you can sit down and breathe some fresh air. If you can manage these things, you should be fine.

13 Hanging Around the House:

Questions About Bed, Bath, and Beyond

"He is happiest, be he king or peasant, who finds peace in his home."—Johann von Goethe

Pregnant women often ask questions about things that otherwise go without a second thought. Drinking a simple glass of tap water can turn into an anxiety-provoking dilemma for some pregnant women. Others find themselves wondering if they should give away a pet cat for the duration of their pregnancy. Many women won't sleep on their backs, afraid to deprive the baby of oxygen. And it's no surprise that women have these worries; almost every day the media reports a new story about something that may be dangerous to pregnant women. This chapter addresses the common questions that pregnant women face, even when they're just "hanging around the house."

Q: *I know I shouldn't sleep on my back but I just can't seem to get comfortable any other way. What risks am I taking by doing this?*

A: None at all. Anyone who suggests that it's dangerous to sleep on your back is talking utter nonsense. Not even the tiniest shred of evidence suggests that sleeping on your back is dangerous. If it were, women would probably have humps. Nature wouldn't leave something as important as a successful pregnancy to chance.

When you lie flat on your back late in pregnancy, the blood flow to the fetus is slightly decreased. On the other hand, when you stand on your head, blood flow to your brain is *increased,* but that doesn't mean standing on your head makes you smarter. Changes in blood flow when you change your position are normal. The baby gets all the blood it needs regardless of your position. Many women do find it uncomfortable to lie on their backs in pregnancy simply because of the size of their belly, but this is a matter of comfort, not safety.

There are some rare cases in which sleeping on your back *might* be best avoided. For example, if the baby has intrauterine growth retardation (a condition in which the baby tends not to get enough oxygen), then it might make sense to avoid lying on your back. But babies don't *get* intrauterine growth retardation from having back-sleeping mothers. It results from chronic problems (like diabetes or high blood pressure) in the mother. In this case, the blood supply is already somewhat compromised so perhaps avoiding lying on your back is a good idea. Otherwise, however you're comfortable is fine.

Q: *I heard my husband should do all the cat litter changing while I'm pregnant. Why is that?*

A: Honestly, there is no good reason for you to avoid cat litter—other than the smell, of course.

The myth that cats should be avoided during pregnancy arose because cats may be infected with toxoplasmosis. Toxoplasmosis is one of the few infections that can pass from mother to baby. Luckily, toxoplasmosis complicates only about one in 10,000 pregnancies in the United States, so in general, it's not worth spending too much time worrying about.

Toxoplasmosis (technically called *toxoplasmosis gondii,* or "toxo" for short) is a parasite with a complex life cycle. People get toxoplasmosis infections from two main sources: undercooked pork and infected soil.

An infected pig or sheep develops cysts in its muscles that contain the toxo parasite. Infected animals then excrete the parasite in their feces. It can remain dormant in the soil for years. Only thorough cooking at high temperatures will destroy these cysts. About half of human toxo infections come from eating undercooked, infected meat.

Most other toxo infections come from oocysts in soil. Oocysts form when cats catch and eat infected animals. An infected cat can excrete oocysts in its droppings. The oocysts remain alive for long periods in soil. Cats are common pets and many have had toxoplasmosis, so it was long assumed that avoiding cats would reduce the risk of toxoplasmosis.

However, recent studies show that cats rarely infect humans directly. Instead, human infection comes from contact with dirt or contaminated water. That is, a neighborhood cat might drop its feces in your garden. These feces may contain oocysts. When you work in the garden, you may touch the oocysts. People may wipe their faces while gardening without washing their hands. This hand-to-mouth contact can lead to toxo infection. On the other hand, people rarely spend hours with their hands in cat litter (and if they do, they have problems far greater than toxoplasmosis infection), and most wash their hands after changing the litter.

Cats probably only shed the toxoplasmosis cysts for a few weeks after they get toxo. Since they only get infected once, infected cats will shed cysts for a short period only *once* during their whole lifetime. After the cysts are shed, it takes several days for them to become infectious. Therefore, if you change the litter daily, you will get rid of any cysts before they are dangerous.

All over the Internet and in pregnancy books, people advise you to avoid cat litter, but this is a lousy way to avoid toxo. The American College of Obstetricians and Gynecologists doesn't recommend this strategy. Infectious disease experts don't recommend it either. These knowledgeable experts recommend thoroughly cooking all meats before eating them, particularly pork and lamb (beef and chicken have not been documented as sources of toxoplasmosis). Some experts also recommend avoiding salami during pregnancy as the toxoplasmosis cysts in pork may not be killed during the curing process.

Most toxo infections come from eating infected meats or from infected soil and water.

Reducing exposure to dirt and water in the environment is harder than cooking meat. But there are things you can do. If you garden, wear gloves. Wash your hands after you have finished. If you've been touching soil, avoid touching your face or mouth or eating without first thoroughly washing your hands.

Q: *Do dogs and other kinds of pets carry infectious diseases like toxoplasmosis?*

A: Cats are the only domestic animal that can carry toxoplasmosis. That is the source of the "stay away from cats" advice. Pigs have a fairly high rate of infection with toxoplasmosis, so don't adopt a pig during your pregnancy. Wild birds can also carry toxoplasmosis so don't capture any wild birds and keep them as pets (birds raised in captivity are safe).

Staying away from pets has never been shown to reduce the incidence of toxoplasmosis during pregnancy. Furthermore, children that are exposed to cats and dogs during the first year of life have fewer allergies as they grow up. So not only are cats and dogs not dangerous, but they might actually improve your family's health!

Q: *What kind of hair coloring products are safe during pregnancy?*

A: None of the thousands of hair care products currently marketed in the United States are dangerous during pregnancy. However, hair care products do not have to undergo rigorous safety testing, but must simply be shown not to be dangerous. Hair product manufacturers don't provide specific information about the effects of their products on pregnancy. But scientists have studied hair treatments like coloring, straightening, and perming and found no risk to pregnancy.

There were some older reports of danger to women who applied hair dyes for more than forty hours a week. Only the busiest cosmetologist will ever be exposed to this quantity of chemicals. Furthermore, later studies showed that even this high of an exposure wasn't risky. If studies of extreme exposures like this demonstrate no risk, then lower exposures (like what you get from having your hair dyed) must be safe.

The bottom line: You can dye your hair!

Q: *Can certain shampoos or soaps be dangerous because of the chemicals in them? Am I safer using "all-natural" products on my skin and hair?*

A: There is absolutely no reason to be concerned about using soaps or shampoos. These products stay on your skin for a very short period of time. And skin's entire function is to keep bad things out. If some soap is absorbed through your skin, the amount is miniscule. Any chemicals absorbed into your bloodstream would be largely blocked by the placenta. Finally, even if such a chemical did get to the fetus, the chance it would cause harm is so small as to be incalculable.

As far as "natural" products go, the only thing that's certain is that they're more expensive than commercial products. If that doesn't bother you, or you like the way they smell or make your skin feel, then by all means use them. Your decision should have nothing to do with trying to reduce risks to your unborn child.

Q: *Is it safe to wear nail polish while I'm pregnant?*

A: Yes, you can wear nail polish throughout pregnancy without worrying. The chemicals used in nail polish can't be absorbed through your nails in any significant amounts. Breathing the fumes from nail polish and nail polish remover, on the other hand, is not a good idea. The organic solvents in these products may be harmful if inhaled for long periods or in enclosed spaces.

You won't breathe in high concentrations of these solvents just painting your nails or removing the nail polish unless you do it in a small, poorly ventilated room. But women who work in nail parlors may be exposed to dangerous levels of these solvents. A study of women with high organic solvent exposure showed an increase in miscarriage compared

Around the House

- Sleep however you're comfortable unless your doctor specifically tells you otherwise.
- Color your hair if it makes you feel good.
- Paint fumes are nasty but they won't hurt your baby. Paint only in well-ventilated areas.

with women who did not have such high exposures. If you work in a setting where you are exposed to fumes from nail polish remover or paint thinner day in and day out, you should seriously consider modifying your exposure for the duration of your pregnancy.

Q: *Are there certain household cleaners, like 409 or Comet, that I should avoid using while I'm pregnant?*

A: No. Cleaning products used in the home *can* be hazardous, but only to *you*, not your unborn child. If being around these products makes you feel ill, or if while cleaning you feel lightheaded, then you are probably being overexposed. If this happens, step outside and have a breath of fresh air.

Exposure to certain cleaning compounds, particularly in combination, can harm your lungs. Your baby, on the other hand, is safe. When you are cleaning, make sure that you open the windows or ventilate the area well. Wear gloves since many cleaning products can irritate the skin (not because they can hurt your baby).

Q: *Should I use a special water filter?*

A: Not unless your water tastes funny. Water filters filter out the large particles that can make water taste bad or look discolored, but they don't filter out smaller particles. Two water contaminants have been suspected of being a risk to pregnant women: trihalomethanes and trichloroethylenes. Studies of these compounds have been somewhat inconclusive, but no clear risk has been found.

Even if these compounds were dangerous, which is far from proven, filtering the water would not remove them. The best way to remove them is simply pour a glass and wait several minutes before drinking it. Many of these chemicals will simply evaporate into the air.

Q: *Is it safe to drink fluoridated water during pregnancy?*

A: Water fluoridation presents no known danger to anybody, pregnant or nonpregnant. Many communities throughout the United States add fluoride to the water to reduce the risk of cavities. The benefits of water fluoridation have been well proven. The risks remain somewhat controversial. Reports that fluoride in water causes Down's syndrome can be found in various books and on several websites. Recently, researchers have concluded that the studies linking fluoridated water and Down's syndrome were so poorly conducted as to be meaningless. Fluoride certainly can be toxic at high doses but these doses are not reached with water fluoridation.

Switching to bottled water "just to be safe" isn't a good idea. First, there is no known risk of drinking fluoridated tap water. Second, there is no reason to think that bottled water is any safer than tap water. Labels with mountain peaks or burbling streams notwithstanding, most bottled water is simply filtered water from some city's water supply. The filtering process only removes particles that affect taste, not contaminants. Furthermore, by law, tap water must be free of infectious organisms, like cryptosporidium, while no such laws apply to bottled water.

U.S. drinking water is extraordinarily safe. In countries where there's no clean drinking water available, the water makes people seriously ill. Our clean water supply may have as much to do with the health of our nation as our medical system does! Unless you are drinking from a well that might be contaminated, you shouldn't worry about drinking from the tap.

Q: *My mother-in-law looks pained whenever I stand in front of the microwave—is this dangerous to my pregnancy?*

A: Not a bit. Here's a bit of explanation of how microwave ovens work: They use very short wavelength ("micro") electromagnetic waves to heat food. These waves are radiation, but not *ionizing* radiation—the type of radiation in X rays. In physics, radiation simply means energy transmitted over a distance. A light bulb, for example, puts out nonionizing radiation in the form of light energy. Microwaves use this kind of nonionizing radiation, unlike the ionizing radiation from X rays, nuclear blasts, or cosmic rays. Ultrasound uses similar nonionizing radiation to "see" a baby through your skin and muscles.

Nonionizing radiation from your microwave oven cannot directly affect the cells in the developing fetus—nor can it affect the cells in your body. Even if you could turn your microwave on with the door open, you couldn't hurt your pregnancy.

There is one way that microwaves could damage a pregnancy, but you'd never be able to get a microwave oven to do it. Microwaves can heat things up (or they wouldn't use them in an oven, right?) and if you were to have a microwave beam directed at you, it could heat you up. If your cells got hot enough, you could be burned. Similarly, if your fetus got hot enough, it could be damaged. This effect would require treatment with enough microwaves to raise your body temperature to near 110 Fahrenheit.

Tell your mother-in-law that unless you actually got inside the microwave and turned it on, there's no way it could hurt you. Microwaves are responsible for some injuries to babies after they're born, however. Some mothers use the microwave to heat up formula or milk. Since microwaves heat things unevenly, one part of the bottle may get to too high a temperature, but drops of milk tested on your wrist may still feel cool. There have been many reports of babies having their mouths or throats scalded as a result. The solution? Either heat the bottle in a pan of warm water, or thoroughly mix the bottle *after* it comes out of the microwave, then test the temperature. If it's warm, but not hot, to the touch, it should be safe.

Q: *Is it safe to paint the baby's room while I'm pregnant?*

A: Absolutely, but you need to use common sense. Work in a well-ventilated room, and take frequent breaks. If you feel faint or light-headed, stop working. Also, be careful climbing ladders; you could injure yourself in a fall.

Paint and paint thinner are not dangerous to pregnant women who are around them only occasionally. For women who are painters by trade, there are some different risks. People who are chronically exposed (and this means daily or nearly daily exposure) to a group of chemicals called organic solvents (paint thinner is one of these solvents) do have an increased risk of malformations in the fetus. But there is *no* increased risk in pregnant women who simply paint a room or two or who spend time in a house that is being painted. For longer exposures, wearing gloves and a well-fitting mask might reduce the danger, although studies to confirm this have not been done.

If your house was painted before 1978, there's a good chance the paint had lead in it. Paint used to be a major source of lead exposure until the federal government outlawed its use. High lead levels during pregnancy may increase fetal problems such as low birth weight and miscarriage, although most lead poisoning comes from children's *direct* exposure to lead, not from prenatal exposure. To protect against lead exposure, just painting over old lead-based paint isn't a good idea. Instead, a professional should examine the paint, determine the lead level, and recommend a plan. There are federal programs to help you make sure the paint in your house is safe. Call the National Lead Information Center at 1-800-424-LEAD for more information.

PART 3

Labor, Delivery, and Postpartum

14 Labor of Love:

Preterm, Term, and Delayed Labor

"Pain is inevitable. Suffering is optional."—M. Kathleen Casey

Labor is the culmination of pregnancy. But labor doesn't always begin when we want, or end the way we want. To many women, there is nothing scarier than hearing the words "preterm labor." Doctors usually don't know what causes a particular woman to go into preterm labor, and even more rarely know how to stop it. For a woman whose doctor suspects preterm labor, this fundamental lack of information can be particularly nerve-racking. Labor can also go wrong by coming not too soon, but too late. "Postterm" pregnancy means a woman is still pregnant two weeks after her due date. When you've spent nearly ten months waiting for something to happen, these two weeks can be agonizing. This chapter provides clear answers to the questions women have about these conditions, explaining preterm, postterm, and complicated labors. The chapter addresses ways doctors deal with abnormal labors, paying specific attention to which treatments work and which don't.

Q: *I started having strong contractions at thirty weeks, should I be worried?*

A: Probably not. It may be hard for you to feel, but your uterus begins to contract regularly after twenty weeks. The important question is whether those contractions are a cause for alarm, or just "practice" for the main event.

The definition of preterm labor as opposed to preterm contractions is that in labor the cervix begins to open. Strong contractions, no matter when they happen, are not labor. On the other hand, contractions, no matter how weak, coupled with dilation or opening of the cervix, are in fact labor.

When you tell your care provider about your contractions, he or she will probably want to examine your cervix. As long as your doctor or midwife feels that your cervix has not dilated, there is no cause for alarm.

Contractions without dilation are often called "Braxton Hicks" contractions. Before the advent of modern pregnancy tests, an English doctor named John Braxton Hicks described a way to determine whether a swelling in the pelvis was an early pregnancy, or a tumor. Braxton Hicks put his hands on a woman's abdomen and carefully felt for rhythmic contractions. If he felt them, he could be sure the swelling was nothing more dangerous than a pregnancy. If there were no contractions, he had to consider whether to operate on the woman to possibly remove a malignant tumor.

We now call any contractions that don't result in dilation (opening) or effacement (thinning) of the cervix "Braxton Hicks" contractions.

Q: *My friend was on bed rest to prevent her contractions from turning into preterm labor. Shouldn't I do that, just to play it safe?*

A: Absolutely not. Bed rest cannot prevent preterm labor; nor is bed rest risk free. Experts agree that most cases of preterm labor can't be prevented—by any method. About one in ten babies is born before thirty-six weeks gestation (the formal definition of "preterm"). More than half of these result from preterm rupture of the amniotic sac, or from infections in the uterus. Currently, these things can't be prevented. Treating uterine infections doesn't stop labor once it's started and there is no way for doctors to "reseal" a broken bag of waters.

Because they can't prevent preterm delivery that result from these more common causes, obstetricians have tried valiantly to slow or stop "idiopathic" preterm labor. Idiopathic preterm labor describes cases where doctors cannot identify an obvious cause of the labor, such as infection.

The best study available study on the topic, funded by a government research agency called the Agency for Healthcare Research and Quality (AHRQ), showed that bed rest added nothing to treatment of preterm labor. Bed rest may be useful in very specific circumstances, particularly for women with a weak or "incompetent" cervix.

That a process as important to the reproduction of the species as labor can't be stopped by changing your position shouldn't really be a surprise. Labor is a powerful force—even with the strongest medications around, doctors can only slow preterm labor by a few days (or weeks at the most). Lying down is pretty weak stuff compared to these medications.

Bed rest is easy to prescribe ("Go home and rest for a while") and makes both doctor and patient feel like something is being done, but it does have a cost. Bed rest, even for forty-eight hours, causes dramatic muscle weakness, leading to pain and other potential problems. And it can be psychologically taxing as well. I've seen countless women hospitalized for bed rest. After about three days most are wishing, either consciously or unconsciously, for labor to start again. Lying down for days on end can literally drive you crazy.

Preterm labor is a serious problem—one that requires serious treatment. If your doctor has determined that you are in labor, and you're more than six weeks from your due date, you should be treated. But treatment should be with things that work—not just things that are easy to do.

Q: *If bed rest doesn't work to stop preterm labor, what does?*

A: There are at least three drugs that can slow it down, but no drugs or treatments effectively stop preterm labor. The drugs used to slow preterm labor are magnesium sulfate, terbutaline, and calcium channel blockers. Each has advantages and disadvantages, but terbutaline is probably the riskiest of the three. The decision about which to use should be left to the team of professionals treating you.

All these medications have risks—including causing heart attacks and lung problems. They should only be given if the expected benefit from delaying delivery by a week or two outweighs this risk. In general, that means they should only be used in pregnancies between twenty-four and thirty-four weeks. Before twenty-four weeks, the chance of delaying delivery long enough to have a baby with even a tiny chance of surviving is small. In this case, taking a dangerous drug has too little upside. Babies born after thirty-four weeks have so few serious problems that the risk of the medications isn't worth taking. In this situation, not taking the drugs has too little downside.

These antilabor drugs should be used for short periods of time only. Many doctors keep women on these medications for weeks, but this is bad practice. The best available evidence clearly shows that giving "maintenance" therapy after preterm labor has stopped has far more risk than benefit.

Q: *Why bother to take potentially dangerous medications at all if they only delay delivery for a week?*

A: Sometimes a week's delay gains a lot, because in that week important things can happen. First, doctors can give a type of medication called a steroid to the mother. Steroids (related to the drugs that body-builders use to "bulk up," but used in much smaller amounts) cross the placenta and accelerate the maturity of the baby's lungs. If every woman who delivered before term got this medicine, the number of babies who had serious problems from prematurity would drop dramatically. Steroids should be given to just about every woman between twenty-four and thirty-four weeks pregnant who gets treatment for preterm labor.

Second, during that week of delay, the mother can be transported to a hospital with experience in caring for preterm babies. Hospitals with Neonatal Intensive Care Units (NICUs) have much better results in caring for these tiny babies than do hospitals without these specialized units.

Q: *I have contractions all the time. I've heard of monitors that you use at home to check contractions. Would that help me catch preterm labor early?*

A: Absolutely not. At least three studies have shown that home uterine activity monitors are worthless in preventing preterm labor. Some doctors still use them, but having you come in for a checkup, or having a nurse call you at home to see how you are doing, works just as well as these devices. These monitors seemed like a big advance when they hit the market. The idea makes sense: Use the monitor to see who is having "too many" contractions, then treat those women to prevent preterm labor. The problem? Not only don't we know what "too many" is, we can't really prevent preterm labor to begin with!

Two things can help predict if you will have preterm labor: ultrasound of the cervix, and a blood test for something called "fetal fibronectin."

The ultrasound works by measuring the length of your cervix. Women with longer cervices have very little risk of preterm delivery. Women with shorter cervices have a higher risk—not high enough that they need to be treated, but that they should be watched more closely.

The fibronectin blood test gives similar information. The level of fetal fibronectin in your blood can help gauge the risk that you will deliver too early. If the test is negative, you can rest easy—the chance of you delivering before term is very low. A positive test is harder to manage, because again, there are no good long-term treatments for preterm labor. At the minimum, a positive test will encourage your doctor to see you more frequently.

Q: *I've heard that epidurals lead to cesarean sections. Is that true?*

A: Not really. Our understanding of the relationship between cesareans and epidurals has evolved somewhat over the years. It's probably true that ten to twenty years ago, epidurals did increase the cesarean delivery rate. But advances in anesthetic techniques over the last decade have lessened this risk. The most recent study shows that there may be one additional cesarean delivery for every forty women who get an epidural.

To give an epidural, an anesthesiologist injects a small amount of medication in the space that surrounds the spinal cord. The medication doesn't reach the spinal cord directly. Very little of it ends up in the mother's bloodstream, so epidurals have long been considered one of the safest forms of pain relief in labor. Without an epidural, pain medication must be given to the mother through an IV. When given IV these drugs reach the baby in fairly high doses. The lung function of babies born to mothers who received IV narcotics in labor can be depressed by the drugs. As a result, these babies are much more likely to need help breathing.

Medications used for an epidural won't affect a baby's breathing, but they can cause extreme relaxation of the mother's pelvic muscles. The pelvic muscles help guide the baby's head into the proper position for delivery. If the muscles are too relaxed, the head may not be positioned properly, increasing the need for a cesarean. To avoid this, more women nowadays get "walking epidurals." A "walking epidural" uses smaller amounts and different combinations of medications, allowing better control over the muscles of the legs and pelvis. Theoretically, a woman can have good enough muscle control to walk around. (In practice, fetal monitoring makes it impractical for most women to walk with a "walking epidural.") Properly done, this type of epidural probably reduces the chance that epidural will lead to cesarean delivery.

To me, a small risk of more cesareans is well worth it, considering how much pain relief an epidural can provide.

Q: *If epidurals are so great, why doesn't everybody have one?*

A: There are downsides to an epidural. It's just that having more cesareans is probably not a major one. Women who have epidurals are more likely to need forceps or vacuum to deliver the baby. For every fifteen women who have an epidural, one additional woman will need vacuum or forceps to aid delivery.

Because of the muscular relaxation an epidural produces, the baby's head may end up in a slightly different position when it comes to the pushing stage of labor. Muscular relaxation from an epidural can also prevent a woman from using her pelvic and abdominal muscles to push in a coordinated way. Since adequate pushing requires strong, coordinated muscular effort, this diminished ability to push can lead to a greater need for "assistance" in the form of vacuum or forceps. (The choice of vacuum or forceps is generally at the physician's discretion since studies have shown these methods to have similar risks and benefits.)

In addition to leading to more "assisted" deliveries, epidurals can make labor a bit longer. The first stage of labor (the dilation stage) lasts about forty-five minutes longer in women who have epidurals. The pushing stage lasts about fifteen minutes longer. If the epidural is given early in labor, it can slow or stop contractions. So, more women who get epidurals also get oxytocin (Pitocin) to keep their labor from slowing too much.

Women who have epidurals are more likely than other women to get mild fevers during labor. It's unclear what causes the fever, but it generally has no impact on the baby. In fact, babies born to mothers who used epidurals are slightly more active at birth than if the mothers used IV medication.

Q: *What about pain? Isn't that the real reason for having an epidural anyway?*

A: When it comes to pain relief, there is little doubt that epidural is superior to other methods. Women who have epidurals have much less pain both during the first stage (dilation) and second stage (pushing) of labor. It's not that there aren't other methods of controlling pain during labor. It's just that epidural controls pain better. In one study, eighty-five percent of the women with epidurals were satisfied with their pain relief, compared to fifty-seven percent of the women who had IV narcotics.

Q: *So, epidural is better?*

A: It's not a matter of better or worse. As with most things, having epidural for anesthesia during labor represents a trade off. Only you can decide whether the trade off is worthwhile. Epidurals provide some of the best pain relief possible and don't increase the risk of cesarean delivery. The use of epidurals does lengthen labor, however, and it increases the need for oxytocin (Pitocin). It also raises the risk that the mother will have a fever in labor.

For most women, the knowledge that their pain will be better relieved, that their babies will be unaffected, and that the risk of cesarean is not dramatically higher tilts them toward wanting an epidural. For others, the increased risk of needing "assistance" with vacuum to deliver the baby, or the idea that their labor will be longer, steers them away from epidural. There is no right or wrong choice.

Q: *My friend developed chronic back pain after her epidural so I'm not sure I want to get one.*

A: I don't think her pain came from the epidural. In the early 1990s, there were reports that women who had epidurals had much greater rates of back pain after delivery. (One study even showed that ten times as many women who had epidurals had back pain.) These early studies were not very well done and more recent studies have disproved this theory. An excellent randomized trial done in England showed that while back pain was very common after delivery, it was no more common among women who had had an epidural than among those who had not.

Q: *I was given Pitocin during my last delivery and had no problems. But I've head many women say it's dangerous. What's the story?*

A: Pitocin (oxytocin) has been used for almost fifty years to increase the strength and frequency of uterine contractions. It is, in many ways, a very powerful and potentially dangerous drug. Before the advent of modern IV dosing pumps, nurses or doctors had to sit by the bedside of a woman getting Pitocin and monitor the number of drops going into her veins. Doctors have learned better ways to use Pitocin and modern electronic IV pumps prevent dangerous overdoses. As a result, this powerful drug has become well understood and can be safely used.

Q: *Why is Pitocin used at all?*

A: In many women, labor starts, then slows or stops. Oxytocin can increase the number and frequency of contractions so that a normal labor begins again. Without it, labor can drag on, a potentially exhausting prospect for the mother and fetus. Longer labor, particularly after the membranes have ruptured, increases the risk of fetal and maternal infection. Pitocin isn't a cure all, but the careful use can prevent some labor problems.

Oxytocin can also help reduce cesarean deliveries. Studies from the United States and Ireland show that giving it when contractions slow can dramatically reduce the cesarean delivery rate. Like most drugs, Pitocin has a good side and a bad side. If properly used, it reduces infections and reduces the cesarean delivery risk. Improperly used, it can be deadly.

Q: *Is it really necessary to have a heart rate monitor on my belly during labor?*

A: Yes and no. The doctors who introduced fetal heart rate monitors had high hopes. They believed that cerebral palsy (a nonprogressive muscular problem) was due largely to trauma or stress suffered during labor and delivery. They hoped that monitoring the fetal heart would allow them to see problems and intervene before injury occurred. Unfortunately, decades of experience with heart rate monitoring have not reduced the cerebral palsy rate.

Hundreds of studies have looked for the benefits of heart rate monitoring. Only one such benefit has been found: Continuous heart rate monitoring reduces the risk that babies will have seizures shortly after birth. The rate of seizures has decreased but, unfortunately, the rate of cerebral palsy has not.

That said, continuous heart rate monitoring has become so common that it is difficult to find doctors who *don't* use it. Other methods of monitoring the baby (either using electronic heart rate monitoring intermittently or listening with a stethoscope) have become so uncommon that most doctors and midwives are not at all skilled with these methods. For this reason alone, electronic fetal heart rate monitoring is here to stay. If you wish to do without it, you need to find a doctor or midwife who has experience monitoring the heart rate using other means. The fetal heart absolutely *must* be monitored to detect important changes in the baby's tolerance of labor. Monitoring does not have to be continuous, as it commonly is in most U.S. hospitals, but monitoring must occur.

Q: *What are internal heart rate monitors and why are they used?*

A: The internal fetal heart rate monitor is a small electrode and wire that clips onto the baby's head. The end of the monitor makes a small cut in the baby's scalp to attach itself securely. The fetal heart rate can be monitored more precisely with an internal monitor than with an external monitor.

But more precise doesn't mean better. Newer, more accurate *external* heart rate monitors are as good as some internal monitors. Internal heart rate monitors should be reserved for special circumstances, for example when the heart rate simply cannot be clearly heard using external monitors. Internal monitoring (both internal contraction monitors and internal heart rate monitors) may slightly increase the risk of uterine infection in labor, and should only be used when there is some potential benefit from them. When the heart rate can be adequately heard with another method, there is no potential benefit.

Q: *What is internal contraction monitoring and why is it used?*

A: An external uterine contraction monitor strapped around the belly identifies when contractions begin and end. External contraction monitoring cannot measure the *strength* of uterine contractions, just their frequency. The internal contraction monitor or *intrauterine pressure catheter* (IUPC) allows accurate measurement of the actual strength of uterine contractions.

This sounds like a terrific innovation, but adds very little to the obstetrician's ability to monitor labor. External monitoring measures contraction frequency perfectly well in most women. Internal monitoring does measure strength of contractions, but this additional information can't really help the obstetrician make better decisions. Studies examining intrauterine pressure catheters have shown that they don't improve labor outcomes.

Why are they in use? Because of the powerful idea that "better measurements must lead to better outcomes." But in the case of internal contraction pressure monitoring, this idea is clearly wrong. Just *feeling* the uterus during contractions can tell the obstetrician whether contractions are strong enough. A doctor can learn just as much by feeling a laboring woman's uterus as by using an internal contraction monitor.

In some very limited circumstances, uterine contractions can't be measured without internal monitors. Very heavy women have so much tissue between the skin and the uterus that an external monitor (or the doctor's hand) just can't tell what's happening.

Internal pressure monitors can also be used to flush water through the uterus. Sometimes, compression of the umbilical cord causes the fetal heart rate to drop dangerously. Flushing water into the uterus will sometimes take pressure off the umbilical cord allowing the baby's heart rate to recover. In general, however, these monitors are unsure and don't add anything to your doctor's ability to monitor labor.

Q: *I'm getting toward my due date and my baby is breech. Am I going to need a cesarean?*

A: You may, but don't give up hope. Once you arrive at the hospital with the baby in breech position, the likelihood is high that you will end up with a cesarean one way or the other. But since you're not quite at your due date yet, there is still time to "turn things around."

The safest way for a baby to be born is vaginally, in a head first direction. So you and your doctor should make some effort to get the baby facing the right way. There are two excellent ways of doing this: one easy to understand and one almost impossible to believe.

The easy-to-understand method involves having you lie in a hospital bed while your obstetrician pushes on the outside of your belly, guiding the baby in a half circle to bring its head pointing down toward the birth canal. This process, called *external cephalic version* (ECV), has been around for many years and has been subject to numerous studies of its safety and success. In experienced hands, ECV can turn a baby head down about half the time.

Rarely, ECV can lead to cesarean delivery, but the benefit of turning the baby around outweighs this small risk. ECV also hurts because it causes a tremendously strong uterine contraction while the baby is being turned. But the pain usually lasts ten to fifteen minutes at the most, and it avoids all the pain associated with a cesarean. ECV is best done around thirty-six weeks. If it's done too much earlier, the baby can spin back to breech again before delivery.

The unbelievable way to turn a breech baby involves a process called *moxibustion,* a traditional Chinese medical procedure. Moxibustion involves burning a plant called *artemisia vulgaris,* or valerian, and using the heat to simulate certain precise points on the body. Moxibustion at a point on the little toe has been *proven* to help turn babies from breech to head down.

In 1998, a randomized controlled trial published in the prestigious *Journal of the American Medical Association* (*JAMA*) *proved* that moxibustion could turn babies to face the right way by the time of delivery. Doctors performed moxibustion beginning at thirty-three weeks of pregnancy in a group of breech babies. In another group, no such procedure was performed. If the baby was still breech at thirty-six weeks, the doctors tried ECV. In the group that had moxibustion plus ECV, almost three-quarters of the babies were head down. In the other group, only half were. Moxibustion and EVC caused no ill effects in any of the babies or mothers.

If a study like this had been done of a pill that could turn babies from breech to head down, you can be sure every woman with a breech baby would be taking it. But Western doctors have so much trouble with the idea that a non-Western technique like moxibustion could work that this procedure has gained very little ground in the United States. Even though we know that vaginal delivery is better than cesarean, and even though this study proved that moxibustion improved the vaginal delivery rate, close-mindedness to nontraditional techniques has condemned thousands of U.S. women to essentially unnecessary cesareans.

In the United States, finding someone who is willing to perform moxibustion might not be easy. Finding someone who does it and works closely with an obstetrician might be close to impossible. Many colleges of Chinese or Oriental medicine may be able to help locate qualified practitioners, as would the American Academy of Medical Acupuncture (see **Resources**). Most Oriental medical doctors (OMDs) would either be able to perform moxibustion or find somebody who can. In the *JAMA* study, doctors watched the babies' heart rates during moxibustion. They never saw any serious heart rate problems, but if you're going to try moxibustion, you should take the same precautions. To do this, you will need both a willing Oriental medical practitioner and a monitoring facility (usually a hospital or doctor's office).

If your baby is breech and you are less than thirty-two weeks, it's worth doing some investigating about both ECV and moxibustion. At the very least, your doctor should be willing to try ECV or refer you to someone who will. ECV is a much better option than cesarean, so it's worth pushing for.

Q: *My doctor tried to do an external cephalic version (ECV), but it didn't work. Do I need a cesarean delivery now?*

A: You probably do. Over the past thirty years, debate has raged among obstetricians about the best way to deliver breech babies. One increasingly vocal school of thought has held that all breech babies should be delivered by cesarean. Another group, concentrated in academic medical centers, has argued the safety of vaginal delivery in certain circumstances. During my training, I learned that performing a vaginal breech delivery was a special skill, a dying art, and I'd be a better obstetrician if I could do it. Two things changed my mind: a personal experience and a large study.

Several years ago, a woman arrived at the hospital in labor with her second child. The baby was breech. This woman was so far along in her labor that I don't know whether we could have done a cesarean even if we wanted to. We decided to wait and try to deliver the baby vaginally. The delivery began well, but after the baby's body delivered, the head got stuck in the birth canal. After several agonizing minutes of maneuvering, we managed to deliver the head. Oxygen had been cut off to the baby's brain for so long that it was born blue and lifeless. Only the vigorous resuscitation efforts by an amazing team of pediatric specialists revived this baby. Even more miraculously, it suffered no injury or harm as a result.

Coincidentally, the same week we delivered this baby, the medical journal *Lancet* published a major study called the Term Breech Trial.

This landmark study of more than 2,000 women established once and for all that cesarean delivery is safer than vaginal delivery for breech babies. Before this study, proponents of cesarean or vaginal delivery each relied on smaller studies that supported their own views. The Term Breech Trial proved that breech babies suffered serious injury or death more frequently if they were born vaginally than if they were delivered by cesarean.

The authors of this study calculated that for every seven breech babies delivered by cesarean, one death or serious complication could be prevented. Compare this to the argument for doing cesareans on babies weighing more than nine pounds (see below), where it would take several *thousand* cesareans to prevent one complication.

The combination of personal experience and this large study has convinced me that vaginal delivery of breech infants no longer has a place in modern obstetrics.

Q: *My doctor wants to do a cesarean at thirty-eight weeks because my baby is getting too big. Is this a good idea?*

A: Probably not. It is true that babies weighing over nine or ten pounds suffer injuries to the nerves in their necks and arms during delivery more than smaller babies do. Big babies break their clavicle during delivery more commonly as well. Finally, the larger the baby, the more likely a cesarean delivery will be needed eventually anyway. With this background, many obstetricians just decide to go directly to cesarean if they think the baby is bigger than nine and a half pounds.

Makes perfect sense, right? Doctors sometimes give the impression that they know exactly how big your baby is at any given time. For example, your ultrasound might say that your baby "weighs nine pounds eight ounces." But even in the best hands, ultrasound can be off by half a pound in either direction. So your doctor's plans are based on faulty information.

The other problem with your doctor's strategy is that the birth injuries he or she's trying to prevent are very rare. For example, the risk of permanent nerve damage to a baby's arm from delivery is less than one out in 300. A study published in the *Journal of the American Med-*

Best Bets for a Safe Labor

- Fetal heart rate monitoring is a must, but it doesn't need to be done throughout labor in low-risk cases.
- "Internal" contraction or heart rate monitoring has few advantages over "external" monitoring.
- Inducing labor because a baby appears to be getting "too big" is generally a bad idea.
- Breech babies should be delivered by cesarean.
- Turning a baby from breech to head down before delivery is safe and may allow a vaginal delivery.
- Epidural is probably the most effective form of pain relief in labor.
- Epidurals probably increase the chance of cesarean delivery.
- Epidurals don't cause long-term back pain.

ical Association (JAMA) showed it would take more than 3,000 cesarean deliveries to prevent one single permanent birth injury. Even worse, those 3,000 cesareans would result in problems of their own—babies can be hurt during cesareans, too.

If there were a better way of knowing which babies would be injured during vaginal delivery, or if we could tell exactly how much a baby was going to weigh, then performing a cesarean would make sense. But we can't. Recommending cesarean for all babies *thought* to be above a certain size results in very little protection at way too high a cost.

Q: *What about just inducing labor at thirty-eight weeks rather than performing a cesarean? Can that make it easier to have a successful vaginal delivery?*

A: Unfortunately not. Many doctors think that inducing labor before the baby is "too big" will reduce the chance of birth injury. The theory behind this makes sense: Bigger babies have more injuries during childbirth. And babies grow as much as half a pound a week toward the end of pregnancy. So, it seems logical that inducing labor before the baby reaches a certain size would reduce the risk of birth injury.

But good theories don't make good medicine. At least a dozen studies have proven that inducing labor to reduce birth injury doesn't work. More inductions didn't lead to fewer injuries in any of the studies. Most of the studies concluded that the only guaranteed results of more inductions was more cesareans. In other words, not only does inducing labor not prevent injury, but it also increases the cesarean rate.

Labor induction isn't always a bad idea: There are times when waiting for normal labor is clearly not smart. For example, if the baby or mother are in danger, any delay can be life threatening. But the strategy of induction to reduce cesarean deliveries and birth injury is a proven failure.

Even worse, many doctors induce labor at thirty-eight weeks because they consider babies born after thirty-eight weeks to be "full term." But inducing labor at thirty-eight weeks can cause problems usually only seen with premature babies. Respiratory distress syndrome (RDS), a common problem among preemies, can occur after thirty-eight weeks. Doctors who suggest induction before thirty-nine weeks without checking the baby's lungs are gambling with your baby's health.

Amniocentesis can easily tell whether the baby's lungs are ready to breathe air. If you haven't had an amniocentesis, your doctor should *never* consider an elective induction before thirty-nine weeks. The American College of Obstetricians and Gynecologists say this very clearly in their guidelines on elective labor induction. Unfortunately, many doctors ignore this advice because the risk of RDS is so low. Your baby's lungs are too important to take even this small risk: Make sure your doctor either waits until thirty-nine weeks or performs an amniocentesis before inducing your labor.

15 The Unkindest Cut of All:

Episiotomies, Cesareans,
Vacuums, and Forceps

"If pregnancy were a book, they would cut the last two chapters."—Nora Ephron

Over the course of her life, a woman is more likely to have an episiotomy or a cesarean delivery than any other procedure or operation. Yet many women feel they don't understand the decision-making process about these procedures very well. Cesareans are done for a wide variety of reasons, some of which can't be assessed until labor is already well underway. On the other hand, there are many situations in which some advance planning and discussion can take place. This chapter answers questions related to the decision to undertake invasive procedures during labor and delivery. It will help clarify the thinking behind these decisions and provide some tips on reducing your chance of having unneeded surgery.

Q: *What's the point of an episiotomy? Should I ask my doctor if she does them?*

A: An episiotomy is a cut made in the vagina to widen the opening through which the baby passes. Many women suffer tears in the vagina during delivery. Episiotomy began as a method for preventing these tears. Doctors thought cutting the vagina was a "cleaner" way of widening it than allowing it to tear naturally. They assumed that cutting the tissues before they stretched out would prevent damage to the vaginal muscles. This muscle damage was thought to be the cause of incontinence (involuntary urine loss). Women who've had children are more likely to develop incontinence, and doctors hoped episiotomies would reduce this risk.

Unfortunately the theory of episiotomies turned out to be wrong. Studies now show that episiotomy should only be performed when necessary (for example, if the baby is in distress and needs to be delivered sooner) and not to prevent future problems. Episiotomy causes more pain, more infections, and more damage to the vagina than do "natural tears." Episiotomy does not reduce the risk of pelvic relaxation later in life. Recent studies have shown that women who go through labor and then have a cesarean delivery have nearly as much incontinence as do women who have vaginal deliveries.

Bottom line: Unless your baby is in distress, your doctor probably should not perform an episiotomy. Good studies prove that episiotomy is not necessary. If your doctor still routinely does them, he or she needs to do some studying. And you need to look for a new doctor.

Q: *My girlfriend had her baby delivered by forceps. Aren't those things against the law by now?*

A: Perhaps amazingly, they are not. Certainly, the use of forceps has dramatically declined over the last thirty years. Before the advent of safe cesarean deliveries, forceps were the only method of delivering babies that were "stuck." Forceps saved many mothers and babies. But if improperly used, forceps can be dangerous.

The first strike against forceps was safe cesareans; the second strike was the invention of the vacuum extractor. Vacuum-assisted delivery involves placing a molded plastic cup on the baby's head and creating a vacuum inside that cup. The obstetrician pulls on the cup, adding some extra force to the mother's pushing efforts.

Vacuums and forceps serve the same purpose, helping deliver babies when the mother's pushing efforts are not enough. Since the vacuum cup is soft plastic, rather than hard metal, many doctors assume it is much safer than forceps. But it's not clear that vacuum is really better than forceps. It is softer and causes fewer tears in the mother's vagina, but it also increases the risk of bleeding inside the baby's eyes and causes more bruising of the baby's scalp.

Researchers have tried to determine which is safer—but they haven't been able to pick a clear winner. Vacuum extractors *look* safer, but looks can be deceiving. Several deaths have been reported with vacuums. Also, they require much less skill to use. And it may be that because they're easy to use, they get overused. No intervention is risk-free—neither vacuum or forceps should be used unless the mother can't push the baby out quickly enough without them.

Q: *Why not just dispense with vacuum and forceps and go with cesarean?*

A: Sometimes, that's exactly the right thing to do. Other times, cesarean might cause more damage to both the mother and the baby. For example, if the mother is really exhausted and can't push the baby the last little bit of the way out, then helping with a vacuum or forceps is less traumatic than performing a cesarean. As in so many things, it's really a matter of judgment. The doctor must have good judgment about when each of these methods is the right way. You can't second-guess your doctor's decisions during your labor since they're made too quickly. The best thing to do is find a doctor whose judgment you trust and let him or her talk you through the decisions that are made throughout labor.

Q: *I had a cesarean with my first baby and I just started talking to my obstetrician about how to deliver the second baby. What advice can you give me?*

A: Obstetricians don't agree about the best way to manage a patient who has had a cesarean in the past. In the final analysis, whether or not to try to delivery vaginally is largely a personal choice that should be guided more by your particular goals and preferences than by anyone else's advice.

In the early days of cesarean delivery, a cut was made on the uterus from top to bottom in order to deliver the baby. These cuts weakened the wall of the uterus and made it prone to tear during labor with subsequent babies. If the uterus does tear during labor, the results can be catastrophic. As a result, "once a cesarean, always a cesarean" became the obstetrician's mantra.

Over the years, obstetricians developed a different type of incision, called a "low transverse incision." This phrase refers not to the location of the skin incision (which confusingly is *also* sometimes called "low transverse" or a "bikini cut") but to the location of the cut on the uterus. This "side to side" incision on the lower part of the uterus heals much better than the older incision type. Better healing dramatically reduces the risk of a ruptured uterus in later labors.

Once the risk of rupturing the uterus goes down, the chances of having a successful vaginal delivery goes up. Against this backdrop, and because of the rising national cesarean delivery rate, most doctors agreed that women should be allowed a "trial of labor" after one cesarean delivery.

"Trial of labor" means that a woman begins labor normally, but gets a cesarean if, during labor, the fetus appears to be in danger. Increasing successful "trials of labor" has been the goal of obstetricians, hospitals, and the American College of Obstetricians and Gynecologists for the last twenty years. After all, if a trial of labor results in a vaginal birth, the difficulty of surgery has been avoided and victory over the rising cesarean delivery rate might be achieved.

As more and more women began to have vaginal deliveries after a first cesarean, scientists studied the actual effects of this policy. At least *fifty* different studies conducted between 1989 and 1999 examined the consequences of a trial of labor compared with a repeat cesarean. Doctors at the University of Michigan Medical School and the University of Toronto examined all fifty of these studies and came to a surprising conclusion: More babies were hurt by allowing trial of labor than by encouraging repeat cesarean delivery. Their conclusions were attacked by many, however, since they did not conduct a new study but rather examined data from many older studies.

Q: *How can I balance all this conflicting information?*

A: In order to help my patients understand that question exactly, I created a computer simulation called a decision analysis. This computer model took account of the potential risks to the mother and baby of a second cesarean delivery. It compared those with the potential risks and benefits of a vaginal delivery. I found that the outcomes from repeat cesarean and trial of labor were so similar that there really was no right answer.

In the computer model, as long as a *vaginal* delivery of a healthy baby was considered to be no better than a cesarean delivery of a healthy baby, cesarean was better. The risks are slightly lower and the benefits slightly higher. However, if a mother feels that having a vaginal delivery is important in and of itself, then trial of labor becomes worthwhile. Skipping a trial of labor and proceeding directly to a second cesarean might reduce the risk of injury to the mother and baby, but this reduction is so tiny that it is easily outweighed if someone places a high value on having a natural birth.

If you don't care one way or another about how your baby is born, then I would recommend going straight to a second cesarean. If you have always wanted to have a vaginal delivery and felt you were denied that opportunity with your first pregnancy, then I would encourage you to have a trial of labor.

Trial of labor results in a vaginal delivery between sixty and eighty percent of the time. As long as you are laboring in a hospital that has an obstetrician and anesthesiologist in the hospital around the clock, the risks of a trial of labor are tiny. If you are planning to deliver in a hospital where the anesthesiologists and obstetricians aren't in the hospital around the clock, then a second cesarean is probably the best way to go. If you are able to find a hospital with an anesthesiologist and obstetrician readily available at all times, then a trial of labor is certainly safe.

Q: *I'm pregnant with my first child and the idea of labor pains just terrify me. Can't I just have a cesarean section from the get go? After all, isn't it true that having a vaginal delivery will cause problems for me later in life?*

A: You raise two points in your question, and both are important to the decision about having a cesarean versus a vaginal delivery. First is the fear of pain. Modern pain relief techniques have truly improved over older methods. Newer techniques for epidural produce remarkable pain relief without interfering with labor. And women report more or less the same amount of pain regardless of how they delivered—cesarean caused more belly pain, but vaginal delivery causes more, well, vaginal pain.

As to your concern about "problems later in life," there really is no hard evidence to support this belief, although common sense suggests it might be true. Problems with involuntary leakage of urine (urinary incontinence) are more common in women who have had vaginal deliveries. Damage to the vaginal canal, including tears and cuts, as well as damage to the muscles around the anus are much more common in women who have vaginal deliveries. But the best studies show that after about six months, women who have had vaginal versus cesarean deliveries have similar rate of problems with incontinence and pain.

So, the evidence is somewhat mixed. Nonetheless, more than thirty percent of female obstetricians say they'd prefer cesarean without first trying to have labor. Female obstetricians clearly believe there might be a long-term benefit in avoiding labor and a vaginal delivery. On the other hand, doctors have been wrong about many things before, so they might be wrong on this too.

Ten years ago, you would have been hard pressed to find a doctor willing to perform a cesarean without any "reason" to do so. Times are changing. More and more obstetricians are being asked this question and more and more are willing to go ahead with a cesarean. In some countries, this phenomenon has been building for years. In Chile, for example, almost forty percent of births are by cesarean. Brazil has a similarly high cesarean delivery rate.

Cesareans can be dangerous and some of the risks are laid out earlier in the chapter. Having a cesarean increases the risk that you have placenta previa and placenta accreta in later pregnancies. In placenta previa, the placenta covers the opening to the uterus, which can result in bleeding during or before labor. In placenta accreta, the placenta has grown abnormally tightly to the uterine wall, which can lead to bleeding and even hysterectomy at the time of cesarean.

There is no easy answer to your question. Pain during labor can be controlled. And it's not clear that a cesarean will reduce your chance of health problems in the long run. In a perfect world, doctors could predict whether your labor would be easy. If it would be, you'd go for it. If it looked like vaginal delivery would be hard, then a cesarean would be the best way to go. Unfortunately, current methods of prediction are not good enough to tell in advance who will have a difficult labor. For the moment, my recommendation is go ahead and try to have a vaginal delivery, but don't be so committed to it that you take unnecessary risks to do so.

Q: *Will having a cesarean delivery reduce the chance that I leak urine when I get older?*

A: Nobody knows, but it might. The more vaginal deliveries a woman has, the more likely she is to leak urine involuntarily later in life. But the problem doesn't usually show up until ten to twenty years later, so it's hard to be sure that deliveries are the cause. Australian researchers found that at six weeks after delivery, three times the number of women who had vaginal deliveries had incontinence as did those who had cesareans. Seems like strong evidence that vaginal delivery causes incontinence, right? But after several months had gone by, most of the cases of incontinence had resolved in both groups. More women who had vaginal deliveries still had it, but the difference was much less dramatic.

A study from Norway published in the *New England Journal of Medicine* in 2003 showed that five or six percent more women had incontinence if they had delivered vaginally compared with by cesarean. They studied 15,000 women and found about twelve percent of those who had vaginal deliveries leaked urine, whereas seven percent of those who had cesareans leaked.

Complete protection against incontinence would probably mean cesarean delivery before labor begins, since the muscles and tissues in the pelvis stretch throughout labor, not just at the moment of birth. A cesarean delivery after twelve hours of labor probably gives less than maximal protection. Research at one university hospital found that one in twelve women who had cesareans without *any* labor had urine leakage after delivery. So even the maximum benefit from cesarean doesn't guarantee the results.

No one knows what the future will bring, but right now there isn't enough proven benefit of cesarean to recommend it over vaginal delivery. It may help reduce incontinence, but major surgery should not be taken lightly. It may turn out that there are long-term benefits from vaginal delivery as well. In the end, only you can decide whether this possible benefit outweighs the risks of surgery.

Q: *I have herpes, so my doctor recommended I have a cesarean. Why is that?*

A: Women with genital herpes can pass it to their child during delivery. *Herpes simplex virus* (HSV) does not cross the placenta, so the fetus is safe during pregnancy. If there is herpes virus in the vagina, the fetus can catch it. Neonatal herpes is very rare, but many babies who get it die.

To prevent this terrible outcome, many doctors recommend a cesarean if the mother has active herpes at the time of delivery. Active herpes means a visible sore on or around the vagina. (Herpes infections in other parts of the body, for example the mouth, do not have any impact on how the baby is delivered.)

This practice of recommending cesarean reduced the transmission of the virus to babies, but it has also greatly increased the cesarean delivery rate. Many women have herpes but very few babies catch it (even if they are delivered vaginally during an outbreak). In other words, it takes thousands of cesareans to prevent one herpes-related death. So, doctors wondered how to reduce the cesarean delivery rate without increasing the risk of neonatal herpes again. It turns out that babies almost never become infected with herpes unless they are born during the mother's very first outbreak of herpes.

If a woman has had herpes for many years and develops an outbreak at the time of delivery, the baby will almost never get infected. During a *first* outbreak, on the other hand, there are many more virus particles in the vagina and a much greater likelihood of infection. Some people have argued that cesarean delivery should be reserved for women who have their *first* outbreak of herpes at the time of delivery. In the Netherlands, this approach has helped to reduce cesareans without increasing the chance of neonatal herpes infections.

Many American doctors are unwilling to change their practice, but a second strategy for reducing cesareans is available. Doctors prescribed a drug called *acyclovir* to women who have herpes. Taken during the last four weeks of pregnancy, acyclovir reduces the risk of a recurrent infection. That is, in women who already have herpes, acyclovir reduces the chance of an outbreak at the time of delivery. No outbreak, no need to consider a cesarean.

Using this strategy to reduce the need for cesareans is becoming more popular but does have its own set of problems. Because neonatal herpes infections are so rare, it's very hard to prove that taking acyclovir reduces the risk of neonatal infection. Acyclovir does reduce the risk of herpes *recurrence*. If the mother has no sores, the doctor will be more comfortable allowing vaginal delivery. Treating herpes with acyclovir in late pregnancy might be a matter of treating the physician more than the mother. Nonetheless, acyclovir appears to be safe during pregnancy and this strategy is probably better than the old method of routine cesarean for everyone with recurrence.

Bottom line: If you have a history of genital herpes, you don't need to *plan* for a cesarean. Your doctor may either watch and wait or treat you with acyclovir. If you have an active sore when you go into labor, he or she will probably recommend a cesarean.

Q: *Isn't cesarean safer than vaginal delivery?*

A: In general, no. Of course, in specific cases, a cesarean is certainly safer. If the baby is in trouble and needs to be delivered quickly, if the pelvis is too small or the baby too big to fit normally, or if the baby is in the breech position, cesarean is the best bet. With multiple pregnancies and certain other less common problems, cesarean may be better. But in the vast majority of cases, vaginal delivery is the way to go.

There might be slightly fewer cases of urinary incontinence in women who have cesarean delivery. However, a cesarean is a major operation.

Cesarean causes more blood loss than does vaginal delivery and leads some women to develop *placenta previa* with later pregnancies. In placenta previa, the placenta lies across the cervix. The placenta can then tear when the cervix begins to dilate, causing massive bleeding. Such bleeding can lead to transfusions and premature delivery. Treating placenta previa sometimes means staying on bed rest for long periods. Serious problems like this are nothing to be trifled with, and the risk of having placenta previa goes up dramatically with each cesarean a woman has.

The risk of an even less common condition called *placenta accreta* increases dramatically with each cesarean as well. In placenta accreta, the placenta grows too tightly to the uterus. At delivery, the placenta doesn't separate from the uterus the way it should, causing severe hemorrhage. Placenta accreta can even lead to hysterectomy. This rare complication is becoming more frequent as the cesarean delivery rate rises.

Cesarean delivery has many benefits in certain circumstances. But the added risks mean that it's not right in every circumstance.

Q: *How much longer does it take to recover from a cesarean than from a vaginal delivery?*

A: Individuals vary so much in their ability to recover after a major stress like labor and delivery (whether vaginal or cesarean) that it's difficult to answer this question. Doctors often say you will be back to normal in about six weeks—they might add one or two weeks for a cesarean. Any woman who's actually *had* a baby will tell you that "six to eight weeks to recover" is nonsense.

Researchers at the Canberra Hospital in Australia confirmed this with a study of more than 1,000 women recovering from vaginal and cesarean deliveries. Sixty percent still felt extremely fatigued two months after vaginal delivery. Half still felt this way after almost six months. At two months, women who had cesareans were more fatigued than were women who had vaginal deliveries, but by four months after delivery both groups felt about the same. The Australian researchers also found that a quarter of women who had vaginal deliveries and a third who had cesareans weren't sleeping well two months after delivery. Again, both groups felt the same by six months.

So women who have cesareans have more fatigue and get less sleep in the first two months after delivery but this resolves by four to six months after delivery. Cesarean delivery causes more abdominal pain (where the scar is) but vaginal delivery causes more pain in the vagina (and they *pay* these researchers to figure this out!). On balance, women have equal amounts of pain from cesarean and vaginal deliveries.

Women in my practice tell me that it takes them six to twelve months to feel normal, however they delivered. Not surprising when you consider how long it took to get to delivery. Ten months worth of pregnancy changes can't be expected to go away overnight. Sad how poorly many obstetricians educate their patients, isn't it? Knowing in advance that almost no one will recover fully after six weeks will keep you from being disappointed when you don't feel better that quickly.

Q: *I desperately want to avoid having a cesarean. Is there anything I can do to reduce my risk?*

A: Yes, there are a few things. First, remember that your ultimate goal is to have a healthy baby and for you to be healthy after the baby is born. While having a vaginal delivery is certainly a worthwhile goal, the introduction of safe cesarean deliveries has reduced the risk of labor to mothers and babies dramatically. In countries that don't have access to cesareans, many more mothers and babies are injured and die during labor than in the United States. That said, you can improve your odds of having a vaginal delivery by taking good care of yourself during your pregnancy.

Staying active throughout your pregnancy will keep you in shape and help you withstand the rigors of labor. Physically fit women have shorter labors, less pain with labor, and fewer cesareans. Physical activity is good for you throughout your life and this means during pregnancy too. If you don't have any medical problems (like heart or lung problems), then you only need a good pair of walking shoes to start exercising.

You should exercise regularly throughout pregnancy. There are no real limits on the amount of exercise you can do, or any arbitrary time

Reducing Your Chance of a Cesarean

Before Pregnancy
- Start exercising regularly.
- Improve your diet (more fresh vegetables and less fat).
- Lose weight if you are overweight.

During Pregnancy
- Continue exercising throughout pregnancy.
- Stick to a healthy diet.
- Choose a doctor who won't jump to do a cesarean.
- Try to stay home until the last minute.*
- Have a trained birth assistant with you during labor.

*Does not apply to women with a history of preterm labor.

at which you should cut back on your exercise, but you do need to listen to your body. During pregnancy, your heart works harder than before pregnancy, so you probably won't be able to do as much as you could before pregnancy. Nonetheless, staying active will keep you healthy and reduce your risk of cesarean.

Eating a healthy diet can also help. Unfortunately, most people in the United States are overweight, including pregnant women. Trying to lose weight during pregnancy isn't smart, but if you want to improve your diet, there's no time like the present. Most American diets are too high in fat and include too many processed foods. They often lack adequate fiber and calcium as well. Eating more whole grains, vegetables, and fruits will help increase your fiber intake while lowering the fat in your diet. Avoiding fast food is a good idea since these heavily processed foods are usually high in sodium and low in fiber. Getting enough calcium by drinking low fat milk can also help balance your diet.

A healthy, balanced diet is an insurance policy against developing gestational diabetes. Less active women and those who gain more weight have a greater risk of diabetes. And women with gestational diabetes have a higher risk of cesarean. This doesn't mean that if you develop diabetes it's your fault, or that you have failed to follow a good enough diet. No strategy is perfect, but having a good diet and staying active will reduce your risk.

Your choice of a doctor can affect your chance of a cesarean. Talk to your doctor early in your pregnancy about how often he or she performs cesareans. Experts don't agree on the "right" rate of cesareans, but many think a rate of ten to fifteen percent is reasonable. Many doctors don't keep careful enough track to give you their exact percentage, but most can give you a general sense of how often they do cesareans.

Even after labor begins, it's not too late to reduce your risk of cesarean. First, stay away from the hospital as long as you can. Hospitals are great places—but not for women in early labor. In early labor, not much can be done for you in the hospital besides giving you pain medication. Pain medication is a great thing, but the sooner you get it, the more it may slow labor. For example, if you have an epidural before your cervix dilates three or four centimeters, your risk of cesarean goes up.

Having a birth assistant with you during your labor can also lower your cesarean risk. Studies have shown that a support person's presence reduces labor pain significantly. It also reduces the risk of forceps, vacuum, and cesarean delivery. Finally, having a support person present has absolutely zero risk. Providing labor support requires no special license, although many of these studies used trained doulas. A doula receives training in the normal progress of labor and in ways to help and support a laboring woman. If you don't want to pay to have an assistant with you during your labor, find a relative or friend who has been through labor (either her own or someone else's).

Eating right, staying active, choosing your doctor carefully, and having a labor support person with you won't guarantee you a vaginal delivery but they will improve your odds. Above all, the most important outcome is that you stay healthy and that your baby comes out healthy—not whether you end up having a cesarean or vaginal delivery.

16 Breast Is Best:

Facts and Myths About Breast-feeding

"My mother never breast fed me. She told me she liked me as a friend."—Rodney Dangerfield.

Over the last several years, after a steady decline, breastfeeding rates have begun to rise. Public awareness campaigns and increasing evidence of the benefits of breastfeeding have probably contributed to this increase. Ultimately, whether to breast-feed or bottle-feed is a personal decision—one that can best be made when the mother is fully informed. Many women wonder what benefits actually come from nursing and how long they must breastfeed before their child gains these benefits. Others wonder what lifestyle changes they might have to make to be able to nurse—whether they have to give up coffee, alcohol, or use a different form of birth control. This chapter addresses the most common questions women ask about the decision to start breastfeeding. It provides a list of things that should be avoided while nursing, and describes some surprising things that don't.

Q: *Isn't there too much hype about breast-feeding? I mean, is bottle-feeding really that bad for a baby?*

A: It's not hype. Breast-feeding is much better. Millions of children who were bottle-fed grow up to be healthy and happy adults, but breast-feeding has numerous advantages. Breast-feeding decreases your baby's risk of ear, lung, and urinary tract infection, and of infectious di-arrhea. Breast-feeding may also decrease the risk of sudden infant death syndrome (SIDS), diabetes, Crohn's disease, and allergies. A system as finely tuned as breast-feeding didn't happen overnight. Evolution has worked for eons to make the perfect food for babies. It shouldn't come as any surprise that man-made alternatives fall short.

Of course, sometimes breast milk isn't best. But in general, it is far superior to formula. It's also much cheaper. Buying a year's worth of in-fant formula costs more than $1,000. Eating enough calories to sustain breast-feeding costs only pennies. And since breast-fed babies get sick less often, there are fewer trips to the pediatrician and fewer missed days from work. All together this spells a clear win for breast-feeding.

Q: *I've heard that breast-feeding reduces your risk of cancer. How could that possibly be true?*

A: Women who breast-feed get fewer ovarian cancers and fewer pre-menopausal breast cancers. This may have to do with changes in hor-mone levels associated with breast-feeding. Breast-feeding reduces estrogen levels and higher levels have been linked to breast cancer. Breast-feeding also keeps you from ovulating. Ovarian cancer risk goes up the more times you ovulate. I don't recommended breast-feeding to reduce ovarian or breast cancer risk, but this possible side benefit is one more reason why "breast is best."

Q: *How long should I breast-feed for? I've heard that if I stop before my baby's three months old, it was a waste.*

A: Nursing for *any* amount of time is better than not nursing, so if you have some reason to need to stop at a particular time, you shouldn't feel guilty that you're not doing enough. One of the most important decisions that you can make after your baby is born is to breast-feed. You should congratulate yourself on doing so.

For some time, pediatricians have been debating the "perfect" length of breast-feeding. They'll probably still be debating it when your child starts college. Researchers at the prestigious Cochrane Collaboration in

Oxford, England found almost 3,000 studies that tried to determine the ideal length of breast-feeding. The studies suggest that it's good to nurse for about six months. But they don't say how much difference every extra week or month makes.

Trust your own judgment to know when to wean. To some women, nursing a baby that can ask to breast-feed in complete sentences seems bizarre. For other women, it's an enjoyable way to stay close to their growing child. It's proof that companies selling formula have done a good job that nursing can still be thought odd despite its many known benefits. At four, one of my children still drank a bottle every night and no one bothered me about it. Had he still been nursing at that age, I'm sure my friends and relatives would have given us no end of grief.

Q: *I have a sinus infection but I don't want to use the antibiotic my doctor prescribed while I'm nursing. What else can I do?*

A: As long as your doctor knows you're nursing, you should probably take the antibiotic. Only a few of the thousands of medications on the market shouldn't be taken while breast-feeding. The only antibiotic doctors usually avoid giving during pregnancy is tetracycline. Taking tetracycline during pregnancy can discolor a baby's teeth. Very little gets through into breast milk, so taking it while nursing is probably safe. It's just not usually given because doctors tend to be overcautious about giving drugs to nursing mothers.

No other antibiotics are known to be dangerous during breast-feeding. In fact, if your baby got a sinus infection, the doctor would possibly prescribe the same antibiotic you're getting. Just treat your sinus infection and continue breast-feeding.

Q: *Why can't I take my regular birth control pills while I'm nursing?*

A: You can take them, it's just a question of when. After a strenuous labor and delivery, it's hard for most of my patients to even imagine having sex again, much less needing to worry about contraception. But getting pregnant less than a year after you deliver increases your risk of pregnancy complications. So, before long you will need to consider con-

Drugs To Avoid While Nursing

- Oxycodone
- Certain antiarthritis drugs (like methotrexate or gold injections)
- Phenindione (a blood thinner)
- Some antidepressants (including doxepin and lithium)
- Phenobarbital
- Tetracycline
- Chloramphenicol
- Most anti-cancer drugs
- Diazepam (Valium)
- The antihypertensive drugs amiodarone and atenolol (propanolol and labetalol are safe)
- Some hormone-containing medications (although birth control pills are safe)
- Drugs that suppress the immune system, like cyclosporin
- Theophylline
- Any radioactive compounds

traception. Most women tend to go back to what has worked for them. In the United States, that usually means birth control pills.

Most women who take birth control pills take the so-called "combined oral contraceptive" (because it combines estrogen and progestin in one pill). The most popular form of birth control in the United States, combined oral contraceptive pills are safe, well tolerated and very effective.

Another type of birth control pill called the progestin only pill ("POP" or "minipill") is less popular. The minipill is less effective than the combined pill and becomes much less effective if pills are skipped or even taken at a different time each day. Nonetheless, it is still an effective contraceptive, just less popular in the United States.

The hormones in birth control pills won't hurt your baby, but they may reduce how much milk you produce. Milk production relies on hormones and birth control pills can dramatically change hormone levels. Birth control pills only affect the *start* of milk production. Once the baby is sucking well and a good milk supply has been established, taking combined oral contraceptives has little effect. To avoid problems with breast-feeding, doctors usually don't suggest restarting combined contraceptives until at least two weeks after delivery.

The second reason not to start combined birth control pills right away is the risk of blood clots. The hormone changes during pregnancy begin to resolve after delivery, but a woman still has an elevated risk of blot clots for about six weeks. Birth control pills increase the risk of blood clots even further. It's safe to start birth control pills after this clotting risk resolves.

If you were happy using combined oral contraceptives before, there's no reason why you can't use them while you're nursing. Just wait until about six weeks after you deliver before starting. If you have been breast-feeding (without formula supplements), you are protected against pregnancy from the day you begin the pills. If you have been supplementing, then you should use a backup method of contraception during the first pill cycle.

Q: *Won't nursing keep me from getting pregnant? Why should I bother with pills at all?*

A: You can prevent pregnancy while nursing using the *lactational amenorrhea method* (LAM). Lactational amenorrhea means "no periods while nursing" (lactation = nursing and amenorrhea = no periods) and works because breast-feeding keeps you from ovulating. Without ovulating, you can't get pregnant. The lactational amenorrhea method has excellent success if (and this is a big if) you breast-feed *exclusively* and frequently. If you supplement with bottles, or if you generally go more than six hours between feedings, then the method doesn't work as well.

This is a great method of birth control, completely natural, and risk free. The one-half to one percent failure rate is about the same as the rate of birth control pill failure. If your baby is more than six months old, or you extend your breast-feeding intervals, the method becomes less reliable.

The lactational amenorrhea method will prevent pregnancy if you can answer no to all three of these questions:

1. Have you had a period since you delivered?

2. Are you supplementing your breast-feeding or going more than four hours during the day or six hours at night between feedings?

3. Is your baby more than six months old?

If you answer no to all three questions you have less than a one in 100 chance of getting pregnant.

Q: *My doctor told me that I should take the "minipill" while I'm nursing. What is that?*

A: The minipill, or progestin only pill, contains only one hormone (progestin) while the combined oral contraceptive contains both estrogen and progestin. Although much less popular in the United States than the combined pill, the progestin minipill works very well. It works in a slightly different way than the combined birth control pill, and as a result gives fewer side effects.

The minipill thickens the mucus in the cervix, preventing sperm from entering the uterus. It also changes the lining of the uterus so the sperm and egg are less likely to implant. Unlike the combined oral contraceptive pill, which prevents ovulation, the minipill only reduces the frequency of ovulation. As a result, the progestin only pill doesn't work as well to control problems related to ovulation (like endometriosis or premenstrual syndrome) but it does prevent pregnancy.

The minipill has no effect on nursing and doesn't increase the risk of blood clotting, so many doctors give women the minipill in the postpartum period. After six weeks, they change to the combined hormone pill.

This strategy works fine, but if you've used the combined oral contraceptive before, it makes more sense just to take nothing for six weeks, then start the combined pill. If you have never used birth control pills, then the progestin only pill is a reasonable way to start. If it's working for you at the end of six weeks, there is no reason to change to a combined pill.

Q: *Besides birth control pills, what can I do for contraception while I'm nursing?*

A: One of the best (and most commonly overlooked) forms of contraception is the IUD. In the United States, IUDs got a bad rap because of the Dalkon shield. The Dalkon IUD's design made it prone to cause uterine infections, some so serious that women died from them. Study after study of the newer IUDs have proven them to be among the safest forms of birth control available. Safer in many ways than birth control pills, which are much more popular.

Current IUDs come in two forms. One releases a small amount of a progesterone-like hormone and the other does not. Both safely and effectively prevent pregnancy. Your doctor can put in your IUD immediately after delivery, eliminating the need for a separate office visit weeks later. Even if you don't get an IUD right after you deliver, you can do it at a postpartum visit. The hormone-releasing IUD reduces menstrual bleeding. Many women love this side effect.

The diaphragm also works perfectly well after delivery. Using one takes practice and learning to use it right after delivery may be tough. If you've used one before, however, there's no reason not to return to it.

Many books recommend that a diaphragm be refitted after each delivery. But if you put your diaphragm in and it doesn't fall out, doesn't hurt, and you can feel that your cervix is covered by the diaphragm (the way you were instructed to do when you first got it), then it's okay to use. Condoms also work perfectly well after delivery.

As you choose a method, keep in mind that most couples have intercourse much less often for the first six months to a year after having a baby. This is completely normal. (If obstetricians mention sex at all, they usually say that it's safe to begin having intercourse six weeks after delivery. But most couples find their sex life takes much longer to return to normal.) You may not want to take birth control pills every day when you're having sex once every six weeks.

Q: *I haven't been drinking coffee during my pregnancy. Now that I'm breast-feeding, can I start again?*

A: You *can* drink coffee during pregnancy and breast-feeding. A small amount of caffeine does cross into breast milk, but caffeine in small amounts doesn't harm babies. In fact, doctors give caffeine to infants to treat sleep apnea (a condition in which the baby fails to breathe normally).

In 1985, a Swiss scientist published a study of infants of mothers who drank up to five cups of coffee a day. The study showed that while a small amount of caffeine did reach the breast milk, it did not affect the infants' heart rates or sleep patterns.

A second study found that even though at five cups of coffee caffeine could be found in the mother's milk, there was none detectable in the baby's bloodstream. At seven cups of coffee, some caffeine could be found in the baby's blood. But even at seven cups, the babies themselves showed no ill effects.

Caffeine won't hurt you and it won't hurt your baby either.

Q: *Can I drink alcohol while I'm breast-feeding?*

A: Most doctors, as well as the American College of Obstetricians and Gynecologists, and the American Academy of Pediatrics, recommend limiting alcohol consumption during breast-feeding. They just don't say what "limiting" means.

Scientists at the Monell Chemical Senses Center in Philadelphia proved that even a small amount of alcohol consumed by the mother changes the taste and odor of breast milk. As a result, a baby whose mother has recently had a drink will suck less vigorously and consume less milk. Fortunately, these effects dissipate quickly. Mothers who nurse more than an hour or two after drinking alcohol won't see these effects.

British researchers recently studied almost 1,000 toddlers to see whether a mother's alcohol use had any effect on development. They found no such effect for women who drink two or fewer drinks a day.

I would certainly avoid drinking in the hour or two before you nurse. Having one or two drinks a day, timed not to interfere with feedings, should be fine.

Q: *How much water or milk do I have to drink when I'm breast-feeding?*

A: One of the most common myths about nursing is that you must drink a certain amount of milk or take other forms of calcium. This is completely untrue. Nursing does make additional demands on your body's calcium. If you don't get enough calcium, the calcium necessary to produce your baby's milk comes from your bones. If you don't replace it, your bones will thin as you age.

Neither you nor your baby will suffer if you don't get enough calcium in your diet—at least in the short run. You need 1,200 to 1,500 milligrams a day of calcium over a lifetime to maintain your bones. You can get this calcium from just about any source—dairy, nondairy, or supplements. If you get less calcium, your risk of osteoporosis goes up year after year. But you are doing your baby absolutely no harm.

The second myth is that you have to drink some preset quantity of fluids to make enough milk. Many new mothers feel guilty if they sit down to nurse without a glass of water next to them. This is just silly. The body has many ways of staying in balance. If you don't drink enough, your kidneys hang on to extra water by concentrating your urine. If that doesn't do it, you'll get thirsty. If you drink enough to keep yourself from being thirsty, you'll make plenty of milk. Only severe dehydration decreases milk production. The belief that you must drink a certain amount of water each day is strictly an urban legend, totally without scientific support.

Q: *Will drinking beer before I nurse increase my milk supply?*

A: It may, but drinking alcohol before you nurse still isn't a good idea. Researchers in Germany who studied this subject found that beer contains a chemical that may increase milk production. But they also found that drinking alcohol before nursing decreases the amount of milk a baby actually drinks. So, beer drinking before nursing might get more milk in your breast, but it won't get more milk to your baby.

The researchers theorized that nonalcoholic beer might increase milk production without decreasing suckling, but that more research was needed.

Q: *The hospital that I'm going to gives out packages for nursing mothers when they're discharged, but the packages include samples of infant formula. Why do they do this?*

A: Companies provide these packages in the hope that they will encourage women to give up nursing. The packaging may say "breast-feeding is best," but the only reason companies pay for these products is because it encourages more women to use formula.

This isn't just my opinion. Nearly a dozen studies show that if you get a discharge package containing formula, you are less likely to be nursing six months later. Why would the companies pay for this stuff if it didn't work? The small benefit of these packages (they usually contain some free items that mothers like) doesn't outweigh their disadvantages. Breast milk is the best milk for a baby. Say no thanks to the package.

Q: *What's with all these lactation consultants? Do I really need them?*

A: Nursing is a natural function and something that almost every mother can do, but support for the breast-feeding mother is crucial. Our society has not made nursing easy. We objectify women's breasts, making it hard for them to nurse in public. We allow companies to give away infant formula to almost every woman in the hospital, and we don't make work life conducive to nursing.

All these factors need a counterbalance. One of the best ways to encourage breast-feeding and to help get yourself on the right track is to get help from someone who knows. You may not need a professional lactation consultant but you should find somebody. Most women get advice from their friends and relatives who have nursed before. Doctors have little or no formal training in advising nursing women, so don't expect too much useful information from them. La Leche League can be a great place to get helpful information and referrals as well.

Q: *Who can answer my questions about nursing, since my pediatrician doesn't seem to have much information?*

A: Unfortunately, breast-feeding, like clinical nutrition, is woefully undertaught in medical school and residency. Friends, relatives, professional lactation consultants, and organizations like the La Leche League (see **Resources**) usually provide much better advice than doctors. But remember when evaluating their advice that there is no one "truth." These people are offering you their opinion. No matter how much experience someone has with nursing, their experience might be different from yours. Don't be disappointed if what they tell you doesn't work. Don't feel guilty if you're not taking their advice. You need to find a way to nurse that works for you. That's the only thing that matters.

Q: *Right after I delivered, the doctor took my baby and placed her on my chest to start nursing. I was kind of shocked by this. Why did he do it?*

A: Nursing right away helps your uterus contract and decreases bleeding. The umbilical cord is usually long enough that it doesn't even need to be cut for you to nurse. Lying skin to skin keeps your baby warm and helps you begin bonding.

Babies are born to nurse. Immediately after they're born, they become wide awake, quiet, and alert. They root around with their mouths and look for something to suckle. In the hospital, nurses or doctors too often place babies on an infant warmer. But you have a built-in baby warmer—your chest.

On the other hand, nursing right away isn't magic. If you don't do it, you haven't lost much. What you do during the first hour won't change your ultimate ability to nurse successfully or your child's development.

Q: *I hate to admit it, but nursing kind of turns me on. Is that normal?*

A: Yes, it is. The sensual and sexual aspects of nursing have been well recognized—it's just that women don't often talk about it. When they discover that nursing sexually arouses them, they feel guilty. Don't worry. These feelings are normal. Enjoy the time you have with your baby. Your feelings don't make you a pervert, they are a normal response to the wonderful thing you're doing.

Q: *What is breast milk jaundice and how do I keep my baby from getting it?*

A: Jaundice is a yellowing of the skin and whites of the eyes. The yellow color results from the breakdown of red blood cells. Breast-fed babies are more likely than bottle-fed babies to develop jaundice. But the whole idea of breast milk jaundice is a little ridiculous. Without bottle-feeding, there would be no breast milk jaundice. What's really happening is that bottle-fed babies fail to develop this *natural* level of jaundice.

Bottle-feeding and blood tests for jaundice both became popular at the same time. Bottle-fed babies have abnormally low values on these tests. From this many doctors concluded that more breast-fed babies suffered from jaundice. Unfortunately, this absurd conclusion has helped steer many women away from breast-feeding.

"Breast milk jaundice" is normal. Not only is it not dangerous, it may be helpful. It's much more likely something abnormal happens when babies are bottle-fed that *keeps* them from developing it. But, since doctors know that extreme jaundice *can* be dangerous, they assumed that even the small amount that comes with breast-feeding might be dangerous as well.

If your baby's skin develops jaundice, your pediatrician might want to check the baby's blood. Doing the test is fine, but rest assured that you won't need to stop breast-feeding to solve the problem. If your baby does develop worrisome jaundice, it's from something *other* than nursing (having a different blood type from the mother can sometimes cause jaundice, for example).

Q: *Is it true that breast-fed babies don't gain enough weight early on?*

A: No, it's not true. What is true is that bottle-fed babies get abnormally fat.

When you go to the pediatrician, he or she weighs and measures your baby and plots that weight and measurement on a piece of graph paper. That graph paper contains a scale describing how "normal" babies grow and develop. In the 1970s, when many of these scales were designed, most American women didn't nurse. As a result, these scales reflect normal growth curves for bottle-fed babies. Bottle-fed babies gain weight too quickly and this is reflected in the growth curves. When you compare a breast-fed baby to these "normal" values, it looks as though the baby is not growing well. The truth is just the reverse.

Bottle-fed babies grow too quickly (which may have undesired consequences down the road). I don't believe it's possible that the natural way to feed your baby would be worse than the man-made way.

Q: *I found a lump in my breast while I was nursing. What should I do?*

A: Don't panic. It's probably nothing more than a clogged milk duct or an early infection. Gently massage the area. Apply a warm compress and nurse more frequently from that side. If the lump stays around for more than a week, visit the doctor.

You need to encourage your doctor to take your finding seriously. I know far too many women who brought a breast lump to their doctor's attention while they were pregnant or immediately after only to have their doctor ignore it. One woman ended up being diagnosed with an invasive breast cancer about a year later. She was treated and happily, six years later, she remains cancer free.

Many doctors don't follow up these lumps in nursing women aggressively enough. If your doctor feels the lump and it does not go away after several weeks, you need a breast biopsy. Only a biopsy can truly identify the cause of the lump. The odds of the lump being cancer are very small. Nonetheless, it needs to be taken seriously.

Q: *Why does one of my breasts keep getting swollen and hot?*

A: You may have mastitis—an infection suffered by almost one in three breast-feeding women. Usually, with continued nursing and antibiotics, the infection resolves quickly. But mastitis can sometimes lead women to stop nursing entirely.

Almost all breast milk has bacteria in it—most of the bacteria come from the skin of the breast or from the baby's mouth. The normal flow of milk out of the breast during nursing keeps the bacteria from building up and causing problems. If milk flow is interrupted, the normal bacteria in the milk can multiply enough to cause infection.

Most women with mastitis have breast pain, muscle or body aches, fever, and chills. The infected breast can be hot, red, and tender. Sometimes, particularly in the first few days after the baby's born, both breasts can get hard and you can develop a low-grade fever. This "breast engorgement fever" is not usually from an infection. Unless one or both breasts become red and tender to the touch, you probably don't have mastitis.

Q: *How do you treat mastitis?*

A: Emptying the infected breast will help fight the infection. The more milk stays inside, the harder it is to fight. Continued nursing poses no risk to the baby. In most cases, the bacteria causing the infection came from the baby's mouth to begin with! All parts of the breast must be emptied to get rid of the bacterial buildup. The best way to do this is by systematically pumping the breast, focusing on getting milk from the top, bottom, left, and right. You can then bottle-feed the baby with the pumped milk. This process alone can get rid of many breast infections.

Most doctors recommend antibiotics as well. The combination of pumping and antibiotics gets rid of the infection faster than either one alone. You should see some improvement within a couple of days of starting treatment, but symptoms can last a week or more.

Q: *I had breast reduction surgery when I was younger, will I still be able to nurse?*

A: It depends on exactly how the surgery was done, but you should at least try. Studies of women who had breast reduction surgery have found that many of them were able to breast-feed. One type of breast reduction leaves the milk ducts attached to the nipple, and if you had this type of surgery, your chances of being able to nurse are higher. In another type of surgery, the nipple and areola are actually moved. This requires cutting the ducts and can make breast-feeding difficult. In any case, there is no harm in trying to nurse. If your baby grows normally, she is getting enough milk.

This is certainly a case where finding a qualified lactation specialist would be helpful (see **Resources**) as most obstetricians have little experience with these situations.

Q: *Can I still nurse if I have breast implants? Does it matter if the implants are silicone or saline?*

A: Many women with breast implants are able to nurse successfully. One determining factor seems to be whether the incision to place the implant was made around or across the areola. Implants placed this way often cut through the milk ducts or damage the nerves necessary to stimulate milk production. Most cosmetic implants are now placed through incisions under the arm. This method doesn't appear to interfere with breast-feeding as much, although some women with implants still cannot breast-feed successfully.

Almost all implants placed in the last decade contain saline (salt water) and there is no reason to think that these implants can change breast milk or affect the baby. Silicone breast implants were removed from general use in 1991, but have recently been reintroduced. Long-term safety concerns aside (there may or may not be an increased risk of some illness in women with silicone implants), some doctors have also expressed concerns about babies nursed by women with these implants. There has been some fear that the silicone, or antibodies to it, could cause problems in babies. These concerns have not been well researched, however. Since breast-feeding has so many known benefits, and the risks of nursing with silicone implants are unknown, attempting to breast-feed if you have silicone implants is a reasonable choice. This is another situation in which consulting with a lactation specialist is a good idea—both to talk about the potential risks, and to get help once you've started to nurse.

Q: *I have inverted nipples, can I breast-feed?*

A: Having inverted or flat nipples can make it more difficult to nurse, but it doesn't make it impossible. Women with inverted nipples are slightly more likely to give up nursing before three months, but most do just fine. Often, nipples that look flat or inverted at the start of pregnancy will protrude outward by delivery. In addition, the baby takes more than just the nipple into its mouth when nursing. By drawing the nipple and areola into its mouth, your baby is able to stimulate milk expression, regardless of the appearance of the nipple. Some lactation specialists recommend nipple shields or cups to draw out the nipple before delivery. These have not been well evaluated, but probably pose little danger if you want to try them.

17 Postpartum Problems:

When Will It All End?

"Lack of patience in small matters can create havoc in great ones."—Chinese Proverb

Delivery may mark the end of pregnancy, but it also marks the beginning of the "postpartum" period. During this time, the changes that allow a baby to grow and develop in the uterus begin to reverse themselves. Hopes for a rapid return to normal are usually misplaced, however. Changes in weight, energy, and sex drive (to name a few things) that took almost a year to develop don't reverse themselves quickly—though they eventually do so. While waiting for normalcy to return, women sometimes develop new problems, ranging from backaches to breast infections to depression. This chapter explains how the body returns to its prepregnancy state and in what time frame. It answers questions about common postpartum problems and how best to treat them.

Q: *It's been six weeks since my delivery, but I still don't feel like having sex. Is this normal?*

A: Yes. A delay of more than six weeks before your sex drive returns is completely normal. Even after six months, many women don't really feel like having sex. And it can be a full year after delivery before couples report a "normal" sex life.

Almost seventy percent of women say that their obstetrician didn't speak to them *at all* about sexuality while they were pregnant, so your concerns are quite understandable. When obstetricians do discuss sex during pregnancy, it's usually about when *not* to have it. For example, women with bleeding or preterm labor commonly hear that they shouldn't have intercourse. Sadly, obstetricians almost never mention the normal ebb and flow of sexual feelings during and after pregnancy.

Sexual urges vary a great deal among women—whether pregnant or not—so generalizing is hard. But most women's interest in sex usually stays the same or drops a little bit in the first trimester. (On the other hand, some couples find the freedom from the need for contraception improves their sex lives.) In the second trimester, many couples have an increase in sexual activity while others have a decrease. Couples generally have sex for the last time until after the baby's born about a month before their due date.

Dr. Kirsten Von Sydow at the University of Hamburg in Germany, an expert in sexuality during pregnancy, studied couples after delivery. She found that one in ten couples had intercourse before their six week checkup. Half had intercourse by six weeks. By the third month postpartum, about ninety percent had sex at least once. The remainder did not begin having intercourse again until seven to thirteen months after delivery.

Not surprisingly, most couples have sex less often in the year after the baby is born. Sheila J., a patient of mine, put it this way, "By the time my bottom stopped being sore and I stopped feeling so exhausted, my baby was already a year old—no wonder we didn't have much sex that year!" Many different studies confirm Sheila's experience: A year after their baby is born, most couples' sex lives have returned to normal. Of course, there is a huge amount of variation in "normal" sexual activity.

It's virtually certain that your sex life will eventually return to normal. Your baby's first year can be a very stressful time; don't let worries about sex overwhelm you. Things will settle down, you will begin to get more sleep and life will become more routine again. When this happens, you will probably find your sex life returning to normal.

Q: *My doctor told me not to have sex until six weeks after delivery. Does that just mean intercourse? Are other forms of sex safe?*

A: Generally speaking, sexual contact other than intercourse is safe before that six week mark, although most women don't feel like having sex of any kind before this. Most obstetricians recommend not having sexual intercourse until either the lochia has stopped or six to eight weeks after birth. This recommendation makes common sense: While you are bleeding you might be more likely to get a vaginal or uterine infection. But oral sex or masturbation shouldn't pose this same risk. There really is no scientific information on these risks, so you should do what seems normal and natural.

Q: *Can't oral sex after delivery be dangerous, or even deadly?*

A: It is true that several women have reportedly died from "air embolism" after delivery. Air embolism occurs when an air bubble forms in the bloodstream then lodges in the brain or lungs. The risk of this extremely rare event may be higher soon after delivery. After delivery, air introduced into the vagina during oral sex may be more easily absorbed into the bloodstream and cause an embolism.

However, it takes quite a bit of air to cause this problem, which probably explains its rarity. During oral sex, very little air actually gets into the vagina. Just remind your partner that the idea is to stimulate you, not to inflate you like a balloon, and you'll be safe.

Q: *We tried to have sex, but it hurt. Will things ever get back to normal?*

A: Yes, things will get back to normal. It just takes time. More than half of women have pain the first time they have intercourse after delivery (even if they've had cesareans). Even six months after delivery, many women still have some pain. And one in three nursing mothers have pain with intercourse. By a year after delivery, the number drops to less than one in ten—about what it is among nonpregnant women.

Q: *Will sex feel different to my husband now that the baby's born?*

A: There is remarkably little information about changes in men's experience of sex after delivery. Women often say their vagina feels "looser" when they return to having sex after delivery. In one study, women reported a return to normal by about three to four months after delivery. Kegel exercises clearly help to reduce a *woman's* sense of looseness—but there's just no good information on whether men notice the change.

Clearly, we could use some better studies on this subject, but sexual enjoyment returns to normal by about six months for most couples.

Q: *I had an episiotomy; will that make it hard to have sex?*

A: It shouldn't. Several studies have found no relationship between having an episiotomy and difficulty with sex. The more severe or the larger the episiotomy, however, the longer it takes to get back to normal. So, things might be slower, but they *will* return to normal.

Surprisingly, the amount of pain you have during labor and complications of labor don't affect postpartum sex very much at all. They may affect your relationship in other ways, however. Difficult or complicated births are stressful for relationships. Sometimes, couples have trouble expressing tenderness toward each other for several months after a traumatic birth. Couples may be so shaken by events that it's hard for them to think about each other the way they did before the birth. This too passes with time—usually no more than a few extra months are needed before things get back on track. If more time has gone by and things still don't feel right, talk to your doctor or a counselor.

Q: *Does having a cesarean make it easier to have sex after delivery?*

A: It does, but not by much. Women who have had cesareans have sex an average of one or two weeks earlier than those who have had vaginal deliveries. They have slightly less pain with intercourse and have a slightly shorter time to resume normal sex lives. These differences are very small when you consider that by six months only half of couples would describe their sex lives as "back to normal."

Q: *When I breast-feed, I feel a very intense arousal that I don't even feel when my husband and I are in bed together. Is this normal?*

A: Almost one-third of women have erotic feelings while nursing. This sexual excitement usually plateaus but some women even have orgasms while nursing.

Sexual arousal while nursing is part of the normal interaction between a nursing mother and her baby. As a society, we generally only see sexual feelings arising between two adults as being acceptable. In truth, these normal sexual feelings occur in other situations. Parents of young children know that children masturbate—sometimes before they can even talk. Erotic feelings while nursing your child are normal; they are not a sign of incest or pedophilia. Think about these feelings in survival terms: The baby "wants" you to feel good about giving it the nourishment and sustenance it needs. In evolutionary terms, these feelings probably helped sustain our species. If nursing didn't feel good, babies would starve. It's probably the same reason sex feels so good—it helps keep the human race going. Don't be afraid of the way nursing makes you feel. You're doing something vital and good—keep it up!

Q: *Does breast-feeding make it hard to have sex?*

A: Yes, it may make sex a bit more difficult. Breast-feeding lowers the body's estrogen level. Less estrogen results in thinner skin lining the vagina, making sex painful. Many of my patients have found that using a lubricant during intercourse makes things more comfortable. Water-based lubricants may be better than oil-based and are less messy. It's also important to slow the process of lovemaking down to allow adequate time for the vagina to lubricate.

Nursing women often say their orgasms are less intense, even though they may have the same degree of sexual enjoyment. Women may leak milk during orgasm and this deters some couples from having sex, but there is no reason to be afraid of this milk discharge. It won't shortchange the baby. As long as you can deal with this slight mess, there's no reason to let it interfere with your sex life.

The longer a woman breast-feeds, the more delay there may be before sexual activity returns to its prepregnancy level. Women who breast-feed for longer tend to enjoy intercourse a little bit less and suffer from slightly more pain during intercourse. When they stop breast-feeding, their frequency of intercourse goes back up. But breast-feeding has many positive effects on the baby's health and you may find that replacing nonsexual contact for sexual intercourse allows you to maintain an intimate relationship without having sex.

Q: Should I circumcise my baby?

A: I honestly have no idea. The pendulum has swung back and forth on the medical benefits of circumcision over the last twenty years. A generation ago, circumcision was recommended to all couples as a way to protect their male children from everything from genital infections to penile cancer. More recent evidence shows that these problems occur equally in circumcised and uncircumcised men.

Circumcision is elective surgery. Not major surgery, but surgery nonetheless. There are two main reasons why couples choose to circumcise their children. First, circumcision may be performed for religious reasons. In most of the world, this is the *only* reason boys are circumcised. In the United States, so many men were circumcised for "hygiene" reasons over the last several decades that many couples now circumcise their boys so they "look like dad."

If you are going to circumcise your baby, you absolutely *must* make sure that the baby receives anesthesia. For many years, doctors theorized that infants felt no pain since their nervous systems were not fully developed. This theory has been *resoundingly* disproved. Babies clearly feel pain with circumcision. And this pain can be reduced with some simple measures. If your doctor says that he or she does circumcisions without anesthesia, find another doctor. This is not a matter to be taken lightly. The research on this point is overwhelming and it's a bad sign if your doctor doesn't "get it."

There are many ways to anesthetize a baby. I recommend using all of them. First, the baby is given a pacifier dipped in sugar water. (The sweetness takes their mind off what's happening down below.) Second, he's given an infant dose of Tylenol just before the procedure. Finally, and most important, a prescription anesthetic is either injected with a very tiny needle into the penis or applied to the skin in thick cream. Putting a needle into the penis certainly sounds like a miserable thing to do, but it's the most effective way to prevent pain during circumcision. The important thing is that your doctor uses *some* type of prescription anesthetic, not what particular type she uses.

Circumcision is a very safe operation with serious complications occurring in less than one in every 1,000 circumcisions. It is still an operation, however, and shouldn't be taken lightly. Understand your own motivations for the operation and make sure your doctor knows how to use at least one of the anesthetic techniques mentioned above.

Q: *My back hurt after delivery. Is this from the epidural?*

A: No. More than half of women have backaches after delivery. Studies have proven that having an epidural doesn't increase your risk. Backaches result from changes in your body during pregnancy, from stress on your lower back from the growing fetus, and from overuse of the muscles during labor. At six months, between forty and fifty percent of women still have backaches. But by a year, most backaches are gone.

If your legs feel numb or if pain shoots down your leg to below your knee, see a doctor before you do anything else. Shooting pains and numbness can be signs of a problem with an intervertebral disc ("slipped disc") and may need other treatment. If your back hurts, but it doesn't radiate to below your knees and your legs aren't numb, some simple things may help.

Postpartum back pain usually comes from irritation of the muscles in the lower back. Stretching and strengthening exercises can go a long way toward relieving this pain, but stretching the back itself usually isn't enough—you need to stretch your leg muscles as well. Begin with slow, gentle toe touches, allowing your upper body to hang down for twenty to thirty seconds at a time—without bouncing. You won't get anywhere *near* your toes the first few times (you may not even see them) but repeat this a minimum of five times a day and you soon will. This stretch works both your lower back and your hamstrings (which often tighten during pregnancy).

The "lunge" stretch helps lengthen the quadriceps muscles—another source of back pain. The quadriceps runs from above the hip to below the knee, so to stretch it requires bending your hip and your knee at the same time. Begin by kneeling on the floor with something at your side to steady yourself on (like a chair or the bed). Put one foot forward (you are down on one knee now), then gently lean your upper body forward until you feel a stretch in the front of your hip. Hold the stretch for twenty to thirty seconds and repeat five times a day.

Beginning a gentle exercise program will also help relieve back pain. Walking is a good way to start if you haven't done much exercise before. Try to reach ten minutes a day, six days a week as your first goal. Babies (even newborns) love the movement of strollers, so this is a great way to tame a cranky infant and reduce your pain at the same time. Gradually increase your walks, aiming for thirty minutes, five times a week.

Finally, you can take aspirin, acetaminophen (Tylenol) or ibuprofen (Motrin, Advil) to relieve the pain and inflammation. These medications are all safe and can be taken while nursing. Your pain *will* go away, so hang in there!

Q: How long before my bottom stops hurting?

A: Some women (very few) have almost no pain after delivery. But the majority have some pain in the vagina or "perineal" area. In about half of women, perineal pain goes away one month after delivery.

Researchers at the University of Sydney in Australia found that twenty percent of women still have pain at two months after delivery. Some still had pain after six months. Women who have episiotomies, as opposed to those who have natural tears, take longer to be pain free.

You should take pain medication as needed to reduce pain after delivery. Tylenol, Advil, aspirin, and prescription drugs like codeine are safe even while nursing. Small amounts of these drugs will cross into the breast milk and may even reach your baby's bloodstream, but these small amounts have no harmful effects. (What do you think they use to treat pain in babies? These exact same drugs!) In the age of modern medicine, you shouldn't suffer unnecessarily.

Q: *What happens to the stitches the doctor used to sew up the tear in my vagina?*

A: They will dissolve. Doctors use one of two kinds of suture material to sew episiotomies. The first, a suture made from sterilized cat gut, dissolves in three to six weeks. The second type, a synthetic suture, dissolves more slowly. Some studies suggest that gut sutures are more irritating and cause more pain than synthetic. On the other hand, synthetic sutures take longer to absorb and can sometimes "hang around" longer than needed. Over the long term, both sutures do the job very well, dissolve when they're no longer needed, and do not cause any significant problems.

Q: *Since my delivery, whenever I cough, I pee a little. Is this ever going to stop?*

A: In almost all cases, this problem resolves, but it can take up to a year. About one in ten women suffers involuntary loss of urine or *postpartum stress incontinence* after delivery. Most commonly, urine leaks when the pressure inside the abdomen increases quickly, for example when you cough, laugh, or sneeze. This increased pressure is the "stress" in "postpartum stress incontinence." Some women also experience "urge incontinence." These women leak when the begin to feel the "urge" to go. Urge incontinence doesn't follow delivery as often as stress incontinence does.

Stress incontinence results from mechanical changes in the position of the bladder and the muscles around the urethra (the tube that carries urine from the bladder to outside the body). And it's not just the strain of delivery that causes these changes. Researchers in the 1980s showed that about eight percent of women who had cesarean deliveries *without having labor* still had stress incontinence after delivery.

However, having a cesarean will lower your risk. In 2003, re-

Kegel Exercises

• After you start to pee, try to contract your muscles and stop your urine stream.

• This may not be possible for the first twenty or thirty attempts. Keep trying. Eventually, you will be able to do it.

• Doing these exercises every time you urinate will quickly recondition the muscles of the vagina.

• Kegel exercises can also reduce the risk of postpartum incontinence.

searchers from Norway showed that having a cesarean cuts your risk of incontinence in half. Their findings, published in the *New England Journal of Medicine*, showed that eight percent of women who had vaginal deliveries had bothersome incontinence, while only four percent of women who had cesareans had the same problem. (They also found that overweight women had more incontinence than any other group, so losing weight is a better way to prevent the problem than having a cesarean.) Perhaps surprisingly, having more or longer tears in the vagina does not increase the risk of incontinence.

By six months, half as many women have troublesome symptoms as did immediately after delivery. Symptoms continue to improve for up to a year after delivery. Doing vaginal exercises (Kegels) speeds up the recovery, while being overweight and smoking significantly slow your recovery. Losing weight and quitting smoking are more important than doing Kegels. But if you can, do all three.

Decades ago, doctors proposed that cutting an episiotomy would prevent stretching of the vaginal muscles during delivery and therefore prevent incontinence. They thought that cutting the muscles, then sewing them back together, would be better than letting them tear. This theory makes some sense, but it turns out to have been a colossal mistake.

Literally millions of women have had episiotomies with the hope that it would prevent incontinence. It doesn't. Over the last ten years, many studies have shown that episiotomy is worthless for preventing postpartum problems. For more on episiotomy, see Chapter 15 , but if your doctor recommends one, you need to seriously consider finding another doctor.

Q: *Since I had my baby, I can't control passing gas anymore; it sometimes just leaks out.*

A: Not being able to control gas and stool after delivery is surprisingly common, but rarely discussed by women or their doctors. Doctors in Israel studied 300 women who had babies in the Lis Maternity Hospital in Tel Aviv and found that one in fifteen could not control passing gas a year after delivery. One in a hundred could not control stool.

If you know fifteen women who've had kids, you probably know at least one who is gas-incontinent. And if you know 100 women who have had kids, you probably know at least one who has had the same problem with her bowel movements. Together, these conditions are called "anal incontinence." Anal incontinence probably comes from injury to the nerves and muscles around the anus. As many as twenty percent of women have some damage to the anal sphincter during vaginal delivery.

Women who have vaginal deliveries have greater risk than those with cesareans, but the risk after cesarean is not zero unless the surgery was done before labor began. Among women who have vaginal deliveries, those who had forceps deliveries are at greater risk. So are those who had episiotomies—yet another reason why the routine use of episiotomy should be abandoned.

Doctors don't agree on the best way to treat anal incontinence. Most specialists recommend waiting several months to see if symptoms resolve spontaneously, as long as an examination and testing of the anal muscles shows no obvious damage. But if the muscles are obviously torn, they should be repaired.

If you are still having these symptoms more than three months after delivery, tell your doctor about it. Don't wait for her to ask you—you may have to wait forever! Your doctor should examine the anal sphincter muscle with specialized pressure testing. If the muscles and nerves are normal, your symptoms will probably go away with time. If you have muscle damage, you should see a specialist about getting it repaired. If incontinence results from nerve damage, there is no clear treatment strategy, but again, seeing a specialist is a good idea.

Q: *Why is my hair falling out?*

A: You may have *postpartum alopecia,* a fancy name for "hair falling out after your baby is born." (This is a classic doctor trick—if you can't treat something effectively, at least give it a Latin name so it *sounds* like you know something about the problem.) Postpartum alopecia usually begins two to five months after delivery. Hair is lost over the entire scalp but baldness never becomes total. I've seen many patients with postpartum alopecia—one who needed a wig until her hair came back—and they all eventually returned to normal.

Hair normally grows in three different cycles. During the "anagen" phase, hair grows rapidly. During "catagen," the hair thickens, and during "telogen," the hair is resting. At the end of telogen, a new hair grows next to the old hair and the old hair begins to fall out. These phases are part of everyone's normal hair cycle. And different hairs are in different parts of the cycle at different times: About eighty-five percent of your hair is in the growth phase, another ten to fifteen percent is in resting phase, and a small percent is in the thickening phase.

After delivery, the hairs can synchronize their phases so that almost all of them are in the resting phase at once. Since at the end of this phase the hair begins to fall out, if many hairs are synchronized, they will all fall out at once. In other words, over the course of a year you would normally lose all this hair anyway, but now all the hair is lost at once.

The falling-out phase can last up to six months and the growing back phase another six to nine months, so it may be a year and a half before things are back to normal. Unfortunately, there are no good treatments other than waiting. In the meantime, see your doctor and get your thyroid level checked, however, since low thyroid can sometimes cause the same problem.

Three to six months after delivery, many women (particularly those who don't have postpartum hair loss) notice that their hair seems fuller or thicker. This same phenomenon of synchronizing hair cycles is responsible. The new hair fullness is notable since almost 100 percent of the hairs are growing rather than the usual eighty-five percent.

While most likely your hair loss simply results from this postpartum synchronization, there are some conditions that should be ruled out other than low thyroid. Iron deficiency can also cause hair loss, but rarely causes *new* hair loss after delivery. Some high blood pressure medications, birth control pills, and some drugs for bipolar disorder or epilepsy can also cause it. If you're not taking any of these medications and your thyroid level is normal, you probably just have to wait for your hair to grow back. Several drugs (both oral medications and medicated rubs or shampoos) have been used to try to speed the hair recovery, although none of them seems to work. Postpartum alopecia is *never* permanent, so waiting it out works fine.

Q: When should I go back to work?

A: For most American women, the decision about when to go back to work is based more on money than on health. The United States provides some of the worst postpartum benefits of any industrialized country. (See **Maternity Leave in Countries Around the World.**)

The Family and Medical Leave Act (FMLA) has been the latest big development in maternity leave, but even this falls short of providing very good benefits. FMLA says that if you have worked for more than a year for a public company or an employer with more than fifty employees, then you have the right to twelve weeks of *unpaid* leave in a twelve-month period for pregnancy, child care, or post pregnancy recovery. If your company has less than fifty employees, or if you work for the government, you're probably not covered by the FMLA. That's right, even though Congress passed the FMLA, they exempted themselves from the law! If you're not covered, your company may still have a policy that permits either paid or unpaid leave, but the limits of the plan are up to them.

FMLA means your job must be waiting when you return. But you may need some money in the meantime, since they don't have to pay you during your leave. State disability insurance may provide some payments. Different states have differing laws about disability leave. During disability leave, you generally get benefits that represent some fraction of your salary. Whether these payments are adequate depends on your personal circumstances.

Doctors will usually certify you as being disabled for at least six weeks after you deliver. The length of private or state payments doesn't always line up with your doctor's certification, though. So, while your doctor might certify you as needing eight weeks of benefits, your company or state disability plan may not provide them.

Q: *How much time off would be ideal?*

A: Experts at the University of Minnesota School of Public Health tried to answer that question. They studied women who took varying amounts of time off from work after childbirth and found that women would be much better off with twenty weeks of leave. That's more than three times what the FMLA provides!

Having twenty weeks off dramatically reduced the number of problems women had when they returned to work. Other experts have found that stress and fatigue increase when women return to the work force too soon.

Maternity Leave in Countries Around the World

- Norway: forty-four weeks at 100 percent pay
- Russia: twenty-eight weeks at 100 percent pay
- Italy: twenty weeks at eighty percent pay
- Chile: eighteen weeks at 100 percent pay
- Canada: eighteen weeks at fifty-five percent pay
- France: sixteen weeks at 100 percent pay
- Germany: fourteen weeks at 100 percent pay
- Japan: fourteen weeks at sixty percent pay
- China: thirteen weeks at 100 percent pay
- United States: twelve weeks unpaid

Adapted from International Labour Organization 1998. Maternity Leave in selected countries

Women whose babies have health problems often suffer high rates of absenteeism from work, making them less productive than they could be. Better maternity benefits would help employers as well as mothers, since women wouldn't be forced back to work before they were ready. Other countries realize this and provide several months of paid maternity leave.

The pathetic benefits in the United States really show how we undervalue women's role as the primary caretaker of small children. This situation is unlikely to change unless there is an organized political movement pressing for these benefits. The best way to get things to change is writing to your Congressperson and voicing your opinion.

Q: *When am I going to stop feeling so exhausted?*

A: When your kids are in college. Actually, I'm not sure if that's true, since my kids are only in middle school. But you'll definitely be tired for the next ten years—I can tell you that from personal experience. The flip side is that you won't need to worry about getting bored for quite some time.

If you're talking about the severe fatigue that comes with pregnancy, you won't have to wait so long for that to go away. Two out of three women feel exhausted two months after delivery. By four months, just over half feel that way. By six months, nearly half of women still feel some fatigue, but less are exhausted.

Taking care of a baby can be an emotional roller coaster and physically demanding. For most parents, however, raising children is also the most rewarding thing they will ever do. This may seem like a meager benefit when you are up with a crying baby at two in the morning, but that does seem to be the basic trade-off.

Q: *What can I do to get my energy back?*

A: First, you should have your doctor check to see whether you are anemic. Anemia, or a low red blood cell count, makes your body work much harder to get oxygen, leaving you feeling weak and worn out. Postpartum anemia is fairly common. The iron your doctor may have prescribed for you after you left the hospital was given precisely to treat anemia.

But if you had excessive bleeding, didn't take the iron, or are a vegetarian, you may still be anemic. If you are, adding iron-rich foods to your diet can help increase your red blood cell count and may help counteract fatigue. Iron-rich foods include organ meats like liver, dark green vegetables like spinach, as well as raisins and lentils.

In a small group of women, abnormal thyroid hormone levels cause fatigue after delivery. If you're exhausted and aren't anemic, talk with your doctor about getting tested for hypothyroidism. This condition af-, fects women far more than men and is easy to treat once it's diagnosed.

By far the most important way to relieve fatigue is to get help. Remember that cliché, "it takes a village to raise a child?" It may be a cliché, but it's true. Women whose husbands or partners help with child care are much less tired. If you don't have a partner, or your partner is unable or unwilling to help, you will need to find other resources. If you are fortunate enough to be able to pay for part-time or full-time help, then of course that can be an excellent option. Single parents may also find help from social services agencies. City and county agencies often provide support services to low-income women.

Many of my patients have parents or in-laws come to visit right after the baby is born. This can be a double-edged sword. Some new parents find this helps them grow closer to their own parents while relieving them of some of the drudgery of caring for a newborn. On the other hand, some grandparents only like to give advice and not to give a hand.

Be assertive in sending nonhelpful people away. Relatives usually give new mothers a fair amount of leeway in their behavior, so you've got a perfect excuse to get rid of the dead wood. Just say you need some time "to bond with your baby." If you hurt any feelings, you can always apologize in a few months, saying that you were so exhausted you didn't know which end was up—not far from the truth anyway.

Taking time off from work can help your energy level. Sadly, the United States has among the worst maternity leave laws of any developed nation. But some companies do provide paid maternity leave. If yours does, take advantage of it. The longer the better.

You should try to sleep whenever you can. Two cardinal rules to help you get enough sleep are: Go to sleep as soon as your baby does, and never wake a sleeping baby.

Healthy, full-term babies have an excellent inborn mechanism for communicating their hunger—it's called crying at the top of their lungs. (If your baby was premature, you *may* need to wake him to nurse.)

Fatigue is nearly unavoidable in the early months after delivery and you need to take a common sense approach to control it. Get as much sleep as you can, eat right, and get help whenever possible. Most women find a dramatic reduction in fatigue over the first few months after delivery, and then a more gradual reduction until finally, after the baby is a year or two old, they feel normal again (and ready to have another baby!).

Q: *Why have I been so sad since my baby was born?*

A: Nobody knows exactly why women often get depressed after childbirth, but being physically weakened, not getting enough sleep, suffering through changes in your relationship with your spouse, and experiencing dramatic changes in your body's hormones play a big part.

Sadness after delivery can range from "postpartum blues," a mild and temporary condition, to postpartum psychosis, a severe psychiatric disorder. As many as eight out of ten postpartum women have postpartum blues. In some sense, this sadness is a normal part of childbirth. You're spent so much time and energy preparing for your child's birth that the actual event can't help being emotionally complex. While you are no doubt overjoyed to have this new child, being a mother is far from simple and can bring many new emotions to the surface.

Remember when you got married? That "joyous" occasional was probably also marked by some moments of sadness if not outright depression. Emotionally charged times are never simple. Being sad doesn't mean you don't love your baby or your husband (even though you might hate both of them occasionally).

Postpartum blues begin within a few days after delivery and peak after about one week. The blues go away after one to two weeks. Women with postpartum blues experience wide mood swings, become easily tearful, and are anxious and irritable. The key feature of postpartum blues is that they don't interfere with your ability to take care of yourself or your baby. Talking through your problems with a supportive friend or relative will help you get through this time. But women who get postpartum blues are at higher risk for developing depression in the first year after their baby is born.

If your baby is less than two weeks old and you feel sad but are still able to care for yourself and your baby, you probably have postpartum blues. You shouldn't need any treatment, but if you're not feeling better by the time your baby is two weeks old, call your doctor. He or she should be able to help decide if what you're experiencing is a normal part of postpartum recovery or something that requires more aggressive treatment. If your obstetrician or family doctor doesn't seem to be able to answer your questions, contact a mental health professional. It's better to call someone and have them reassure you than fail to call and lengthen your suffering.

Q: *I'm so sad I can hardly get out of bed. Are you sure that's normal?*

A: Being that sad is *not* normal—you may be clinically depressed. Depression differs from the postpartum blues in many ways. Postpartum blues go away on their own, depression usually requires treatment. The blues don't keep you in bed all day, nor will they keep you from taking care of your baby or yourself. Depression can make it impossible even to do the simplest tasks. Depression is a serious illness that needs to be treated aggressively to get good results.

Very few obstetricians do a good enough job of checking to see if their patients are depressed. Many women go months before a doctor finally realizes that they have an illness that requires treatment. Make no mistake, depression is an *illness*—just like diabetes or high blood pressure. It absolutely must be treated.

The first step toward treatment is a proper diagnosis. Because obstetricians seldom have enough training to cope with postpartum depression, you should take charge of diagnosing yourself. The accompanying table provides a ten-question test called the Edinburgh Postnatal Depression Scale. Read these questions and score your answers as shown. Contact your doctor immediately if you have an abnormal score.

True postpartum depression usually doesn't begin until three to six months after the baby is born. Unexplained sadness, guilt feelings, inability to concentrate, insomnia, and loss of appetite are the most common symptoms. Women with postpartum depression often feel that they can't care for their baby. And while many women with postpartum depression *think* about harming their children, it is extremely rare for them to do it.

Many women see these depressive symptoms as signs that they are

The Edinburgh Postnatal Depression Scale

Check the answer that applies to how you have felt over the past seven days, not just today.

1. I have been able to laugh and see the funny side of things
    - ❑ as much as I always could
    - ❑ not quite as much as now
    - ❑ definitely not so much now
    - ❑ not at all

2. I have looked forward with enjoyment to things
    - ❑ as much as I ever did
    - ❑ rather less than I used to
    - ❑ definitely not so much now
    - ❑ not at all

3. I have blamed myself unnecessarily when things went wrong
    - ❑ most of the time
    - ❑ some of the time
    - ❑ not very often
    - ❑ never

4. I have been anxious or worried for no good reason
    - ❑ not at all
    - ❑ hardly ever
    - ❑ sometimes
    - ❑ very often

5. I have felt quite scared or panicky for no good reason
    - ❑ quite a lot
    - ❑ sometimes
    - ❑ not much
    - ❑ not at all

6. Things have been getting on top of me
    - ❑ most of the time I haven't been able to cope at all
    - ❑ sometimes I haven't been able to been coping as well as usual
    - ❑ most of the time I have coped quite well
    - ❑ I have been coping as well as ever

7. I have been so unhappy that I have difficulty sleeping
❑   most of the time
❑   sometimes
❑   not very often
❑   not at all

8. I have felt sad or miserable
❑   most of the time
❑   quite often
❑   not very often
❑   not at all

9. I have been so unhappy that I've been crying
❑   most of the time
❑   quite often
❑   only occasionally
❑   not at all

10. The thought of harming myself has occurred to me
❑   quite often
❑   sometimes
❑   hardly ever
❑   never

Scoring: If you answered anything other than never on the last question, you should talk to your doctor immediately. Otherwise, the test is scored by assigning a point value to each answer. For questions 1, 2, and 4, 0 is given to the first answer, 1 to the second, 2 to the third, and 3 to the fourth. For the other questions, 3 is given for the first answer, 2 for the second, 1 for the third, and 0 for the fourth. Add all the points together. If your score is 12 or more, or if you scored greater than 0 on question 10, you should contact your doctor immediately.

bad mothers. This can add to guilt feelings and worsen the depressive symptoms. In truth, a depressed woman is no more "responsible" for her difficulty in caring for her child than a woman who has breast cancer is responsible for that. Illnesses, whether medical or psychiatric, are not our fault. They are simply illnesses that need to be treated.

Q: *Won't my depression just go away on its own?*

A: No. Postpartum depression rarely gets better on its own. While it's important to treat all depression, treating postpartum depression may be even more important. Newborns may suffer long-term effects if their mothers are depressed. The earlier treatment begins, the more rapid and more easily full recovery is achieved.

Sadly, many doctors withhold treatment, mistakenly believing that postpartum depression will go away on its own. Depression after the first month or two of a baby's life is *by definition* not postpartum blues, and is not normal. Delaying treatment, or taking a wait-and-see approach once depression has been diagnosed is not smart.

Treatment of postpartum depression involves providing social support, psychotherapy, and drug treatment. Many national and international groups provide support for women with postpartum depression, and these groups are often a good place to start when seeking treatment. Psychotherapy by a trained professional, whether psychiatrist, psychologist or counselor can help. Drug treatment may be added to, or used instead of, psychotherapy.

Q: *My doctor prescribed antidepressants for my postpartum depression. Shouldn't I wait to take the medication until I'm done nursing?*

A: Definitely not. Drug treatment should not be withheld because of nursing. The risk of not treating postpartum depression is so great, and the risks so small, that withholding treatment in this situation makes no sense.

You should discuss your specific antidepresssant medication with your pediatrician, but in general there are no known serious risks from taking antidepressants while nursing, although some medications (like Prozac) may cause stomach upset in babies whose mothers nurse while taking those drugs. The known benefits of both drug treatment for depression and of nursing are so large that they outweigh any theoretical risks from the medication.

Resources

ORGANIZATIONS
Agency for Healthcare Research and Quality
540 Gaither Road
Rockville, MD 20850
(301) 427-1364
Email: info@ahrq.gov
http://www.ahcpr.gov/

American Association of Colleges of Osteopathic Medicine
5550 Friendship Blvd., Suite 310
Chevy Chase, MD 20815-7231
Fax: (301) 968-4101
http://www.aacom.org

American Academy of Medical Acupuncture
4929 Wilshire Boulevard
Suite 428
Los Angeles, California 90010
(323) 937-5514
Email: JDOWDEN@prodigy.net
http://www.medicalacupuncture.org/

American College of Nurse-Midwives
818 Connecticut Avenue, NW, Suite 900
Washington, DC 20006
Phone: 202-728-9860
Fax: 202-728-9897
http://www.midwife.org

American College of Obstetricians and Gynecologists
409 12th St., SW, PO Box 96920
Washington, DC 20090
http://www.acog.com

American Dietetic Association
(312) 899-0040
http://www.eatright.org

Centers for Disease Control and Prevention
1600 Clifton Rd.
Atlanta, GA 30333
Phone: (800) 311-3435
http://www.cdc.gov

Center for Evaluation of Risks to Human Reproduction
Phone: (510) 597-1393
Fax: (510) 597-1399
http://www.cehn.org/cehn/resourceguide/cfteorc.html

Center for Food Safety and Applied Nutrition
5100 Paint Branch Parkway
College Park, MD 20740-3835

Environmental Protection Agency
Ariel Rios Building
1200 Pennsylvania Avenue, NW
Washington, DC 20460
(202) 272-0167
http://www.epa.gov

Federal Aviation Administration
800 Independence Ave., SW
Washington, DC 20591
http://www2.faa.gov/utilities/contactus.cfm

Federation of State Medical Boards of the United States, Inc.
PO Box 619850

Dallas, TX 75261-9850
Phone: (817) 868-4000
Fax: (817) 868-4099
Federation Credentials Verification Service: fcvs@fsmb.org
http://www.fsmb.org

Food and Drug Administration
5600 Fishers Lane
Rockville, MD 20857
Phone: 888-INFO-FDA
http://www.fda.gov

Motherisk
Medication safety phone line
(416) 813-678
Nausea and Vomiting of Pregnancy Helpline
(800) 436-8477
Alcohol and Substance Use Helpline
(877) 327-4636
http://www.motherisk.org

National Headache Foundation
Phone: (888) NHF-5552
http://www.headaches.org

Occupational Health and Safety Administration
200 Constitution Avenue, NW
Washington, DC 20210
Phone: 1-800-321-OSHA (6742)
http://www.osha.gov/

Organization of Teratology Information Services (OTIS)
Phone: (888) 285-3410
http://www.otispregnancy.org

Royal College of Obstetricians and Gynecologists
27 Sussex Place, Regent's Park, London NW1 4RG
Phone: +44 (0)20 7772 6200
Fax: +44 (0)20 7723 0575
http://www.rcog.org.uk/

U.S. Department of State
2201 C Street, NW
Washington, DC 20520
Hotline for American Travelers:
202-647-5225
http://www.state.gov

U.S. Nuclear Regulatory Commission
Washington, DC 20555
Phone: 800-368-5642
http://www.nrc.gov

Useful phone numbers and Web sites
National Lead Information Center
(800) 424-LEAD
http://www.epa.gov/opptintr/lead/

American Association of Poison Control Centers
800-222-1222
http://www.aapcc.org

Doulas
http://doulanetwork.com/

La Leche League
1400 N. Meacham Road
Schaumburg, IL 60173-4808
(847) 519-7730
http://www.lalecheleague.org/

Books
Clapp, JF. *Exercising Through Your Pregnancy.* Addicus Books. 2002.

Goodwin, C., and M. Broder. *What Your Doctor May Not Tell You About Fibroids.* Warner Books. 2003.

Blumenthal, Mark and Josef Brinckman (eds.)
Herbal Medicine: Expanded Commission E Monographs. Integrative Medicine Communication, 2000.

Glossary

Abortion Medical term for a pregnancy that ends before twenty weeks of gestation. Induced abortion is performed by a physician. Spontaneous abortion happens on its own (commonly called *miscarriage*).

Acetaminophen Generic name for the active ingredient in Tylenol. Reduces pain. Can be safely used in pregnancy, but recommended dose (4,000 milligrams in twenty-four hours) should not be exceeded.

Acupressure Technique similar to acupuncture, but points are stimulated with firm pressure, rather than needles.

Acupuncture Ancient technique of inserting very thin needles into certain key points on the body in order to treat diseases.

Amalgam Mixture of materials commonly used to fill cavities in teeth. Amalgams release a small amount of mercury vapor over time. Mercury is toxic in large amounts, so placing this type of filling during pregnancy is not recommended.

Amniocentesis (amnio) An invasive test in which a needle is passed through the abdominal wall into the amniotic sac. Commonly used to examine the baby's chromosomes.

Amniotic sac The fluid-filled sac that contains the developing fetus. This sac acts as a cushion, protecting the fetus from injury. Amniotic fluid comes from both fetal urine and from the developing lungs.

Anemia Low red blood cell count. Some degree of anemia is normal in pregnancy. Greater than normal drops in red blood cell count can lead to maternal fatigue or slow fetal growth and may need to be treated.

Antihistamine Class of medications that reduce the release of the chemical called histamine from cells. Antihistamines are sold both as allergy medications and as sleep aids. The antihistamine doxylamine can be used to treat nausea in pregnancy.

Antiphospholipid antibody syndrome Condition in which a person forms antibodies to portions of his or her own body. In rare cases may be a cause of recurrent miscarriage.

APGAR score The Apgar scoring system provides a standardized means by which the baby's condition is assessed at birth. Signs rated are skin color, muscle tone, breathing attempts, heartbeat, and response to stimulus, such as a touch or a pin-prick. Babies are rated twice, immediately after birth and five minutes later, because many babies, especially anesthetized ones, take some time to turn pink and to begin full breathing on their own.

Asthma Disease of the lungs in which the air passages are abnormally sensitive to irritants. When these irritants reach the lungs, they cause narrowing of the air passages. Untreated asthma can be life threatening. Asthma should be aggressively treated during pregnancy, since constricting the air passages reduces the flow of oxygen to the fetus.

Biofeedback Process of converting certain brainwaves to sound or light. Used to train people to control bodily processes (like heart rate) that are not usually under conscious control.

Birth defect Physical abnormality present at birth. Minor birth defects occur in about one out of every thirty births.

Braxton Hicks contractions Rhythmic contractions of the uterus that do not lead to labor. These contractions are commonly felt after twenty weeks of pregnancy. They do not indicate preterm labor.

Calcium channel blockers Class of drugs used to treat high blood pressure. These drugs may also be used to slow preterm labor.

Carbon monoxide Colorless and odorless gas that can be poisonous. Contained in cigarette smoke. Carbon monoxide in the blood prevents red blood cells from carrying oxygen.

Carpal tunnel syndrome Nerve problem in which the nerves leading to the hand are compressed. Produces pain and tingling in the fingers. May occur during pregnancy and resolve after delivery.

Chorionic villus sampling (CVS) An invasive test in which cells from outside the amniotic sac are used to examine the baby's chromosomes. The cells are obtained by passing a tube through the vagina, past the cervix, and to the outside of the amniotic sac.

Chromosomes Strands of DNA that contain the "roadmap" for creating a person. People normally have forty-six chromosomes (twenty-three pairs). If a developing embryo is missing all or part of a chromosome, miscarriage or developmental abnormalities can result.

Crohn's disease Disease of the intestines, also called inflammatory bowel disease. Symptoms may include fever and abdominal pain.

CT scan Computed Tomography. A test used to create an image of internal organs using X rays and a computer to assemble images.

Cytomegalovirus (CMV) Virus in the same family as the virus that causes herpes. Generally causes no symptoms in children or adults, but can cause fetal effects if mother is infected during pregnancy.

Diabetes Illness in which the body either fails to produce, or doesn't respond normally to, insulin. Results in higher-than-normal blood sugar levels. During pregnancy, diabetes can lead to abnormal growth, with babies that are too big or too small (depending on the type of diabetes and how long it has been present).

Doula Trained birth assistant. Training is not necessarily formal or associated with certification, but involves understanding normal labor and how to support a laboring woman.

Down's syndrome Also called Trisomy 21. A condition in which there are three, rather than the normal two, copies of chromosome 21. Produces various abnormalities including lower-than-normal intelligence and a characteristic facial appearance.

Echinacea Herbal supplement that may shorten the length of colds. Appears to be safe during pregnancy.

Eclampsia Seizure associated with pregnancy. Preventing eclampsia is considered one of the main goals of identifying women with preeclampsia.

Electrolytes Chemicals that are present in normal bodily fluids. The proper balance of electrolytes is necessary for normal functioning. Diarrhea, vomiting, and dehydration may cause electrolyte imbalances.

Embryo Early stages of a developing organism, broadly used to refer to stages immediately following fertilization of an egg through implantation and very early pregnancy (i.e., from conception to the eighth week of pregnancy).

Epidural Method of giving anesthetic by injecting it into the area just outside the spinal cord. Currently the most popular form of pain relief in labor in the United States. Epidural can effectively relieve pain but is not without side effects, one of which is slightly increased cesarean delivery rate.

Epilepsy Disease in which abnormal electric discharges in the brain cause seizures—involuntary muscular and brain activity.

Episiotomy Cut made in the back part of the vagina during delivery. The theory that cutting an episiotomy is better than the natural tearing that can happen during delivery has been proved wrong.

External cephalic version (ECV) Process of turning a baby from breech to head down position using pressure on the outside of the mother's abdomen.

Fallopian tubes The narrow tubes that connect the ovaries and the uterus. Fertilization of the egg by the sperm usually occurs in the fallopian tubes.

Family and Medical Leave Act (FMLA) Act of Congress requiring large employers to provide twelve weeks of unpaid leave for childbirth or other significant events. Does not apply to all employers.

Fertilization Uniting of egg and sperm, which produces an embryo. Occurs in the fallopian tube.

Fetal alcohol syndrome Series of birth defects that are linked to heavy alcohol use during pregnancy. Complicates about one in five hundred births.

Fetus Unborn baby; from about seven to eight weeks of development until birth. Prior to that time considered an embryo.

Fibroid Benign (not cancerous) growth in the uterus. More than half of women have at least one fibroid by age forty. Fibroids may sometimes cause fertility problems or difficulty during pregnancy.

Folic acid (folate) Nutrient that must be present in the diet in small amounts to allow normal bodily functioning. Women who do not get enough folic acid have a higher risk of having a child whose spinal cord does not form correctly (spina bifida). Folic acid is now added to cereals and breads in the United States in order to lower the risk of these spinal cord problems.

Genes Portions of chromosomes that contain the "road map" that tells the body how to make or do certain things. A single gene may be responsible for something as simple as eye color or as complex as preventing breast cancer.

Growth retardation Abnormally slow growth of the developing fetus. Also called *intrauterine growth retardation* (IUGR). May be caused by a variety of illnesses or conditions that restrict the flow of oxygen or nutrients to the fetus.

HCG *Human chorionic gonadotrophin*. A hormone released by the fertilized egg and placenta. This is the most common hormone looked for by pregnancy tests.

Hepatitis Liver infection or inflammation. There are many infectious organisms that cause hepatitis. Different types of hepatitis are transmitted in different ways: hepatitis A often comes from seafood, whereas hepatitis C may be sexually transmitted.

Hyperemesis gravidarum Medical term for severe nausea and vomiting in pregnancy. Women with this condition are frequently hospitalized and require intravenous fluids and nutrition. Can often be treated with medications.

Hypertension High blood pressure. Blood pressure above 120/80 is now considered to be high. May occur during pregnancy as part of preeclampsia.

Ibuprofen Generic name for the active ingredient in Advil and Motrin. Reduces pain and inflammation. Can be used to treat aches and pains in pregnancy, but should not be used long term.

Implantation The name for the attachment of an embryo to the lining of the uterus. Before implantation, most substances in the mother's bloodstream cannot reach the embryo.

In vitro Latin for "in glass." Used in medicine to refer to something that occurs or is tested outside the body. During in vitro fertilization, the egg and sperm unite in a laboratory environment, not in the body.

In vivo Latin for "in the living." Used to refer to tests or processes that occur inside the body.

Incontinence Involuntary loss of urine. In pregnant women, most commonly occurs when coughing or laughing and is experienced by nearly half of pregnant women during the third trimester. Generally resolves without treatment after delivery.

Intrauterine growth retardation (IUGR) See growth retardation.

Intrauterine pressure catheter (IUPC) Plastic tube that can be passed through the cervix and into the uterus during delivery to measure the strength of uterine contractions. Can also be used to fill the uterus with fluid to prevent compression of the umbilical cord during delivery.

Ionizing radiation Radiation, such as X rays and gamma rays (high energy photons), that causes atoms to release electrons and become ions. Biologically significant radiation is an ionizing dose of radiation above 155 electron volts, which may have carcinogenic, mutagenic, or teratogenic health effects in humans.

Kegel exercises Exercises designed to strengthen the muscles of the vagina and pelvis. These exercises speed recovery from postpartum incontinence.

Lactational amenorrhea method (LAM) Birth control technique for mothers who are breast-feeding without supplementing with formula. Relies on breast-feeding's natural ability to suppress ovulation.

Listeria Infection caused by a bacteria called *Listeria monocytogenes*. Infection during pregnancy can lead to miscarriage. Infection is spread through contaminated food.

Macrosomia Term used to describe a baby that is above the normal range of size at birth. These babies are more likely to be delivered by cesarean, but recognizing macrosomia before delivery is not always possible. Literally means "big body."

Magnesium sulfate Chemical compound used to prevent the seizures associated with preeclampsia. May also protect babies from cerebral palsy.

Mastitis Inflammation and infection of the breast. Usually occurs when a milk duct is plugged and bacteria within the breast multiply. Treated with warm compresses, continued nursing, and antibiotics.

Midwife—nurse, lay Birth assistant. Nurse midwives are typically trained nurses first who go through a certification process involving classroom and hands-on training. Lay midwives have no formal training.

Migraine Severe and often debilitating headache. Tendency to have migraines runs in families. Migraines may worsen during pregnancy.

Moxibustion Traditional Chinese medical practice of burning valerian root near certain points on the body. When performed at the proper points, has been shown to improve the chance of a breech baby turning to the head-down position.

MRI Magnetic resonance imaging. A test used to examine internal organs. It produces a picture of these organs by measuring changes in cells when they are exposed to a magnetic field.

National Practioner Data Bank Federal database of actions against medical professionals designed to prevent doctors who have lost their license in one state from moving to another without begin found out. Cannot be used by individuals to search for information on their doctor.

Organic solvents Group of chemicals with many industrial uses. Also found in nail polish remover and paint thinner. Extensive exposure, or exposure in inadequately ventilated areas, can be dangerous during pregnancy.

Osteopath (DO) Physician whose training tends to focus on treating the whole patient, rather than signs or symptoms of one disease. These medical practioners have all the privileges of medical doctors (e.g., they can write prescriptions, perform surgery if trained to do so, etc).

Ovulation The release of an egg from the ovary. Usually occurs every month, with the egg being released from one ovary one month and the other ovary the following month.

Oxytocin (Pitocin) Hormone medication that can be given to start labor or to increase uterine contractions after labor has started. Its use must be carefully monitored by trained nurses since high doses can be dangerous.

Parvovirus Family of viruses. Most commonly discussed member of this family is parvovirus B19, a virus that can cause fever and rash in children. Can severely affect a fetus if the mother is infected during pregnancy.

Pasteurization Process of rapidly heating milk to very high temperatures. Kills harmful bacteria and retards spoilage.

Phenylketonuria (PKU) Rare hereditary condition in which the amino acid phenylalanine is not properly metabolized. It can cause severe mental retardation if not treated. Can be easily detected by a blood test. Most states require a screening test for all newborns, generally done with a heelstick shortly after birth.

Phonophobia Latin for "fear of sound." Describes the sensitivity to sound that sometimes accompanies migraine headaches.

Photophobia Latin for "fear of light." Used to describe sensitivity or pain when seeing light. Occurs with some migraines.

Phthalates Chemical byproduct of plastics that may leak into food or liquids. There has been suspicion that these chemicals cause harmful effects, but no proof of these effects has been found.

Placenta accreta Condition in which the placenta grows abnormally tightly into the wall of the uterus and, at delivery remains stuck to the uterus, causing excessive bleeding. Surgery is sometimes needed to remove it.

Placenta previa Condition in which the placenta lies across the cervix. The cervix, or opening to the uterus, is normally unobstructed, since the baby must pass through it to be born. Placenta previa may resolve on its own, but if it does not, cesarean delivery is necessary.

Polycystic ovary syndrome (PCOS) "Poly" means many, so polycystic means many cysts. A relatively common cause of difficulty getting pregnant, PCOS occurs when an egg fails to grow to maturity each month. Instead, many small, immature eggs remain in the ovary. Each egg lies in a small sac, or cyst, which gives the condition its name.

Postpartum alopecia Hair loss following delivery. Never leads to total baldness and always returns to normal. Usually begins three to six months after delivery.

Postpartum blues Sadness and letdown that follows delivery. Most women experience this and it resolves without treatment by one to two weeks after delivery.

Postpartum depression Sadness that can follow delivery, particularly in women with a history of depression. Usually begins several months after delivery. Associated with extreme sadness, loss of appetite, insomnia, and feelings of being a poor mother. Postpartum depression requires medical treatment and does not resolve on its own.

Postpartum psychosis Affects about one in 1,000 postpartum women. This rare form of postpartum depression is more likely to occur in women who have bipolar disorder, schizophrenia, or a family member who has experienced these diseases. Onset is sudden and usually occurs within the first two to three weeks after delivery. Symptoms may include hallucinations, delusions, severe insomnia, extreme anxiety and agitation, suicidal or homicidal thoughts, and/or bizarre feelings and behavior. Postpartum psychosis requires medical treatment.

Preeclampsia Condition in which blood pressure is elevated and protein appears in the urine during pregnancy. A small number of women who have preeclampsia will develop seizures before, during, or after delivery. There is no known treatment for preeclampsia other than delivery. Checking blood pressure and testing the urine for protein at each prenatal visit helps identify this condition as early as possible.

Pulmonary embolism Formation of a blood clot in the veins which then travels to the lungs. In young women, it is more likely to occur during pregnancy than outside of pregnancy, but it is still extremely rare.

Qi, yin, yang In Chinese philosophy and religion, two principles one negative (yin) and one positive (yang). The relationship of any contrasting pair: female-male as well as cold-hot, wet-dry, weak-strong, etc. A balance of yin and yang is considered to be essential to health. A deficiency of either can lead to disease. Qi or Chi (pronounced chee) is a difficult concept to translate. It's usually left untranslated because there is no single English word that conveys all parts of the Chinese concept. The word that comes closest is energy.

Randomized trial Type of medical study in which the participants are divided between two treatments by a chance event, like a coin flip. This kind of study is considered the ideal way to determine which of two treatments yields better results.

Rectus diastasis Gap between the two strong, straplike abdominal muscles that often widens during pregnancy. Doing sit-ups does not worsen this gap.

Relaxin Hormone released during pregnancy that may be responsible for some of the physical changes, such as widening of the rectus diastasis, or softening of the joint between the pubic bones, that occur during pregnancy.

Repetitive strain injury Injuries that result from performing the same physical activities over and over. May affect workers on assembly lines as well as frequent typists or others who engage in repetitive activity.

Respiratory distress syndrome (RDS) Lung condition that affects premature babies more than full term ones.

Ruptured membranes Breaking of the amniotic sac around the fetus. Since the sac provides protection against the outside world, after the membranes have ruptured, the baby faces a higher risk of infection.

Shingles A reactivation of a previous varicella virus infection.

Sudden infant death syndrome (SIDS) Rare, unexplained death of newborn infants. Risk can be reduced significantly by placing babies on their backs to sleep.

Terbutaline Medication used to slow preterm labor. Vastly overused in the United States, this drug has significant side effects ranging from bothersome (fast heartbeat) to serious (heart attack).

Thermoregulation Process by which the body controls its own temperature. Allows body temperature to remain constant at about 98.6 degrees, regardless of the temperature outside.

Toxoplasmosis Infection caused by a parasite called *toxoplasma gondii*. Occurs in about one in 10,000 pregnancies. Most commonly spread by eating undercooked pork.

Trihalomethanes (THM) A byproduct of water chlorination. There is some evidence of increased risk of miscarriage in women who drink water with high THM levels. Can be removed from water by allowing the water to stand for one minute after it comes from the tap.

Ultrasound Test commonly used to examine the developing fetus. Uses high frequency sound waves to form a picture. There are no known risks of ultrasound and it can demonstrate many physical abnormalities.

Varicella Zoster Also called "varicella." Virus responsible for chicken pox.

Bibliography

CHAPTER ONE

Agarwal, S.K., and A.F. Haney. "Does recommending timed intercourse really help the infertile couple?" *Obstetrics and Gynecology* 84 (August 1994): 307–10.

Axmon, A., L. Rylander, U. Stromberg, E. Dyremark, and L. Hagmar. "Polychlorinated biphenyls in blood plasma among Swedish female fish consumers in relation to time to pregnancy." *Journal of Toxicology and Environmental Health* 64 (November 2001): 485–98.

Barbieri, R.L. "The initial fertility consultation: recommendations concerning cigarette smoking, body mass index, and alcohol and caffeine consumption." *American Journal of Obstetrics and Gynecology* 185 (Nov 2001): 1168–73.

Caan B., C.P. Quesenberry, Jr, and A.O. Coates. "Differences in fertility associated with caffeinated beverage consumption." *American Journal of Public Health* 88 (Feb 1998): 270–4.

Chasan-Taber, L., W.C. Willett, M.J. Stampfer, D. Spiegelman, B.A. Rosner, D.J. Hunter, G.A. Colditz, and J.E. Manson. "Oral contraceptives and ovulatory causes of delayed fertility." *American Journal of Epidemiology* 146 (Aug 1997): 258–65.

Clark, A.M., B. Thornley, L. Tomlinson, C. Galletley, and R.J. Norman. "Weight loss in obese infertile women results in improvement in reproductive outcome for all forms of fertility treatment." *Human Reproduction* 13 (Jun 1998): 1502–5.

Doll, H., M. Vessey, and R. Painter. "Return of fertility in nulliparous women after discontinuation of the intrauterine device: comparison with women discontinuing other methods of contraception." *British Journal of Obstetrics and Gynecology* 108 (March 2001): 305–14.

Dunson, D.B., D.D. Baird, A.J. Wilcox, and C.R. Weinberg. "Day-specific probabilities of clinical pregnancy based on two studies with imperfect measures of ovulation." *Human Reproduction* 14 (July 1999): 1835–9.

Dunson, D.B., B. Colombo, and D.D. Baird. "Changes with age in the level and duration of fertility in the menstrual cycle." *Human Reproduction* 17 (May 2002): 1399–1403.

Ferreira-Poblete, A. "The probability of conception on different days of the cycle with respect to ovulation: an overview." *Advances in Contraception* 13 (Jun–Sep 1997): 83–95.

Fiscella, K., H.J. Kitzman, R.E. Cole, D. Sidora, and D. Olds. "Delayed first pregnancy among African-American adolescent smokers." *Journal of Adolescent Health* 23 (Oct 1998): 232–7.

Ford, W.C., K. North, H. Taylor, A. Farrow, M.G. Hull, J. Golding, and the ASLPAC Study Team. "Increasing paternal age is associated with delayed conception in a large population of fertile couples: evidence for declining fecundity in men." *Human Reproduction* 15 (Aug 2000): 1703–8.

Frisch, R.E. "Body fat, menarche, fitness and fertility." *Human Reproduction* 2 (Aug 1987): 521–33.

Hakim, R.B., R.H. Gray, and H. Zacur. "Alcohol and caffeine consumption and decreased fertility." *Fertility and Sterility* 70 (Oct. 1998): 632–7.

Hawkes, W.C., and P.J. Turek. "Effects of dietary selenium on sperm motility in healthy men." *Journal of Andrology* 22 (Sept–Oct 2001): 764–72.

Hjollund, N.H., T.K. Jensen, J.P. Bonde, T.B. Henriksen, A.M. Andersson, H.A. Kolstad, E. Ernst, A. Giwercman, N.E. Skakkebaek, and J. Olsen. "Distress and reduced fertility: a follow-up study of first-pregnancy planners." *Fertility and Sterility* 72 (July 1999): 47–53.

Humfrey, C.D. "Phytoestrogens and human health effects: weighing up the current evidence." *Natural Toxins* 6 (May 1998): 51–9.

James, W.H. "Sex ratio, coital rate, hormones and time of fertilization within the cycle." *Annals of Human Biology* 24 (Sept–Oct 1997): 403–9.

Jensen, T.K., T.B. Henriksen, N.H. Hjollund, T. Scheike, H. Kolstad, A. Giwercman, E. Ernst, J.P. Bonde, N.E. Skakkebaek, and J. Olson. "Caffeine intake and fecundability: a follow-up study among 430 Danish couples planning their first pregnancy." *Reproductive Toxicology* 12 (May–Jun 1998): 289–95.

Jensen, T.K., N.H. Hjollund, T.B. Henriksen, T. Scheike, H. Kolstad, A. Giwercman, E. Ernst, J.P. Bonde, N.E. Skakkebaek, and J. Olsen. "Does moderate alcohol consumption affect fertility? Follow up study among couples planning first pregnancy." *British Medical Journal* 317 (Aug 1998): 505–10.

Johnson, N., P. Vandekerckhove, A. Watson, R. Lilford, T. Harada, and E. Hughes. "Tubal flushing for subfertility" (Cochrane Review). In: *The Cochrane Library,* Issue 3, 2002. Chichester, UK: John Wiley & Sons Ltd.

Katz, J., K.P. West, Jr., S.K. Khatry, E.K. Pradhan, S.C. LeClerq, P. Christian, L.S. Wu, R.K. Adhikari, S.R. Shrestha, and A. Sommer. "Maternal low-dose vitamin A or beta-carotene supplementation has no effect on fetal loss and early infant mortality: a randomized cluster trial in Nepal." *American Journal of Clinical Nutrition* 71 (June 2000): 1570–6.

Kidd, S.A., B. Eskenazi, and A.J. Wyrobek. "Effects of male age on semen quality and fertility: a review of the literature." *Fertility and Sterility* 75 (Feb 2001): 237–48.

Krey, L., H. Liu, J. Zhang, and J. Grifo. "Fertility and maternal age: strategies to improve pregnancy outcome." *Annals of the New York Academy of Sciences* 943 (Sep 2001): 26–33.

Meacham, R.B., and M.J. Murray. "Reproductive function in the aging male." *The Urologic Clinics of North America* 21 (Aug 1994): 549–56.

Paulus, W.E., M. Zhang, E. Strehler, I. El-Danasouri, and K. Sterzik. "Influence of acupuncture on the pregnancy rate in patients who undergo assisted reproduction therapy." *Fertility and Sterility* 77 (April 2002): 721–4.

Rozati, R., P.P. Reddy, P. Reddanna, and R. Mujtaba. "Xenoestrogens and male infertility: myth or reality?" *Asian Journal of Andrology* 2 (Dec 2002): 263–9.

Rush, D. "Nutritional services during pregnancy and birthweight: a retrospective matched pair analysis." *Canadian Medical Association Journal* 125 (Sept 1981): 567–76.

Sauer, M.V. "The impact of age on reproductive potential: lessons learned from oocyte donation." *Maturitas* 30 (Oct 1998): 221–5.

Sills, E.S., I. Kirman, S.S. Thatcher III, and G.D. Palermo. "Sex-selection of human spermatozoa: evolution of current techniques and applications." *Archives of Gynecology and Obstetrics* 261 (Jun 1998): 109–15.

Speroff, L. "The effects of oral contraceptives on reproduction." *International Journal of Fertility* 34 Suppl (1989): 34–9.

Stanford, J.B., G.L. White, and H. Hatasaka. "Timing intercourse to achieve pregnancy: current evidence." *Obstetrics and Gynecology* 100 (Dec 2002): 1333–41.

Torfs, C.P., P.L. Lam, D.M. Schaffer, and R.J. Brand. "Association between mothers' nutrient intake and their offspring's risk of gastroschisis." *Teratology* 58 (Dec 1998): 241–50.

Van Wezel-Meijler, G., and J.M. Wit. "The offspring of mothers with anorexia nervosa: a high risk group for undernutrition and stunting?" *European Journal of Pediatrics* 149 (Nov 1989): 130–5.

Vine, M.F. "Smoking and male reproduction: a review." *International Journal of Andrology* 19 (Dec 1996): 323–7.

CHAPTER TWO

The American College of Obstetricians and Gynecologists. "Guidelines for Diagnostic Imaging During Pregnancy." ACOG Committee Opinion Number 158. September 1995. Published by ACOG Washington D.C.

"Accutane and Pregnancy." *Organization of Teratology Information Services.* July 2000. http://www.otispregnancy.org/.

Bove, F., Y. Shim, and P. Zeitz. "Drinking water contaminants and adverse pregnancy outcomes: a review." *Environmental Health Perspectives* 110 Suppl 1 (Feb 2002): 61–74.

Cramer, D.W., and L.A. Wise. "The epidemiology of recurrent pregnancy loss." *Seminars in Reproductive Medicine* 18 (2000): 331–9.

Damilakis, J., K. Perisinakis, P. Prassopoulos, E. Dimovasili, H. Varveris, and N. Gourtsoyiannis. "Conceptus radiation dose and risk from chest screen-film radiography." *European Radiology* 13 (Feb 2003): 406–12.

Goldstein, R.R., M.S. Croughan, and P.A. Robertson. "Neonatal outcomes in immediate versus delayed conceptions after spontaneous abortion: a retrospective case series." *American Journal of Obstetrics and Gynecology* 186 (Jun 2002): 1230–6.

Henriet, L., and M. Kaminski. "Impact of induced abortions on subsequent pregnancy outcome: the 1995 French national perinatal survey." *British Journal of Obstetrics and Gynaecology* 108 (Oct 2001): 1036–42.

"Home pregnancy tests reviewed." Bandolier 1999. http://www.jr2.ox.ac.uk/bandolier/band64/b64-7.html/.

La Vecchia, C., and A. Tavani. "Epidemiological evidence on hair dyes and the risk of cancer in humans." *European Journal of Cancer Prevention* 4 (Feb 1995): 31–43.

Latka, M., J. Kline, and M. Hatch. "Exercise and spontaneous abortion of known karyotype." *Epidemiology* 10 (Jan 1999): 73–5.

Olshan, A.F., N.E. Breslow, J.M. Falletta, S. Grufferman, T. Pendergrass, L. Robison, M. Waskerwitz, E.G. Woods, T.J. Vietti, and G.D. Hammond. "Risk factors for Wilms tumor. Report from the National Wilms Tumor Study." *Cancer* 72 (Aug 1993): 938–44.

Sharara, F.I., D.B. Seifer, J.A. Flaws. "Environmental toxicants and female reproduction." *Fertility and Sterility* 70 (Oct 1998): 613–22.

Swan, S.H., K. Waller, B. Hopkins, G. Windham, L. Fenster, C. Schaefer, and R.R. Neutra. "A prospective study of spontaneous abortion: relation to amount and source of drinking water consumed in early pregnancy." *Epidemiology* 9 (Mar 1998): 126–33.

Wilcox, A.J., D.D. Baird, D. Dunson, R. McChesney, and C.R. Weinberg. "Natural limits of pregnancy testing in relation to the expected menstrual period." *Journal of the American Medical Association* 286 (Oct 2001): 1759–61.

Wilson, P.D., C.A. Loffredo, A. Correa-Villasenor, and C. Ferencz. "Attributable fraction for cardiac malformations." *American Journal of Epidemiology* 148 (Sep 1998): 414–23.

CHAPTER THREE

"Basic Facts About Certified Nurse-Midwives." *American College of Nurse-Midwives,* 2002. http://www.midwife.org/prof/displan.cfm?id+6/.

The National Practitioner Data Bank-Healthcare Integrity and Protection Data Bank (NPDB-HIPDB). September 2001. http://www.npdh-hipdb.com/.

United Nations Department of Economic and Social Affairs. Statistics Division. Millennium Indicators. 2003. http://millenniumindicators.un.org/unsd/mi/mi.asp/.

CHAPTER FOUR

Belew, C. "Herbs and the childbearing woman." *Journal of Nurse-Midwifery* 44 (May/June 1999): 231–52.

Center for the Evaluation of Risks to Human Reproduction: X-ray Radiation. *U.S. National Institutes of Health.* May 13, 2002. http://cerhr.niehs.nih.gov/genpub/topics/x_ray-ccae.html/.

"Complementary medicines and the common cold." National Prescribing Service Limited. http://www.nps.org.au

"Consumer Labs claims 44 percent of echinacea products failed testing." May 7, 2001. Virgo Publishing Inc. http://www.herbs.org/current/clabechin.htm

Dashe, J.S., and L.C. Gilstrap. "Antibiotic use in pregnancy." *Obstetrics and Gynecology Clinics* 24 (Sept 1997): 617–29.

"Dental care during pregnancy." British Dental Association Briefing, May 1998.

"Embryo Dose From Maternal Diagnostic X-Ray Examinations." Government of British Columbia Ministry of Health Services. http://www.healthservices.gov.bc.ca/rpteb/rhpp/embryo01.html/.

Gallo, M., M. Sarkar, W. Au, K. Pietrzak, B. Comas, M. Smith, T.V. Jaeger, A. Einarson, and G. Koren. "Pregnancy outcome following gestational exposure to echinacea." *Archives of Internal Medicine* 160 (Nov 2000): 3141–3.

"Guidelines for Diagnostic Imaging During Pregnancy." *ACOG Committee Opinion, Number 158*. September 1995.

Hofmeyr, G.J., A.N. Atallah, and L. Duley. "Calcium supplementation during pregnancy for preventing hypertensive disorders and related problems" (Cochrane Review). In: *The Cochrane Library*, Issue 1, 2004. Chichester, UK: John Wiley & Sons, Ltd.

"How Does Radiation Affect the Public." *U.S. Nuclear Regulatory Commission*. September 23, 2002. http://www.nrc.gov/what-we-eo/radiation/affect.html/.

Kaptchuk, T.J. "Acupuncture: theory, efficacy, and practice." *Annals of Internal Medicine* 136 (March 2002): 374–83.

Koren, G. "Antihistamines are safe during the first trimester." *Motherisk*. January 1997. http://www.motherisk.org/updates/jan97.php3/.

Mahomed, K. "Iron and folate supplementation in pregnancy" (Cochrane Review). In: *The Cochrane Library*, Issue 1, 2004. Chichester, UK: John Wiley & Sons, Ltd.

Marcus, D.A. "Focus on primary care: diagnosis and management of headache in women." *Obstetrical and Gynecological Survey* 54 (Jun 1999): 95–402.

Marcus, D.A., L. Scharff, and D.C. Turk. "Nonpharmacological management of headaches during pregnancy." *Psychosomatic Medicine* 57 (Nov–Dec 1995): 527–35.

Paulson, G.W. "Headaches in women, including women who are pregnant." *American Journal of Obstetrics and Gynecology* 173 (Dec 1995):1734–41.

"Precautionary advice for Dentists and Pregnant Women." *Ministry of Health*. July 27, 1999. http://www.moh.govt.nz/moh.nsf/0/d64e946aafa0c6f14c2567bb000b852a?OpenDocument/.

Rader, J.I., and E.A. Yetley. "Nationwide folate fortification has complex ramifications and requires careful monitoring over time." *Archives of Internal Medicine* 162 (March 2002): 608–9.

Scharff, L., D.A. Marcus, and D.C. Turk. "Headache during pregnancy in the postpartum: a prospective study." *Headache* 37 (Apr 1997): 203–10.

Silberstein, S.D. "Migraine and pregnancy." *Neurologic Clinics* 15 (1997): 209–31.

"Snots' Corner—Cold Remedies." *Bandolier Library*. October 1996. http://www.jr2.ox.ac.uk/bandolier/band32/b32-7.html/.

Wedenberg, K., B. Moen, and A. Norling. "A prospective randomized study comparing acupuncture with physiotherapy for low-back and pelvic pain in pregnancy." *Acta Obstetricia et Gynecologica Scandinavica* 79 (May 2000): 331–5.

Young, G., and D. Jewell. "Interventions for preventing and treating pelvic and back pain in pregnancy" (Cochrane Review). In: *The Cochrane Library*, Issue 1, 2004. Chichester, UK: John Wiley & Sons, Ltd.

Von Wald, T., and A.D. Walling. "Headache During Pregnancy." *Obstetrical and Gynecological Survey* 57 (Mar 2002): 179–85.

Wantke, F., M. Gotz, and R. Jarisch. "Histamine-free diet: treatment of choice for histamine-induced food intolerance and supporting treatment for chronic headaches." *Clinical and Experimental Allergy* 23 (Dec 1993): 982–5.

CHAPTER FIVE

"Drug of Choice for Morning Sickness." *Motherisk*. 2001. http://www.motherisk.org/drugs/morntxt.php3/.

Erdem, A., M. Arslan, M. Erdem, G. Yildirim, and O. Himmetoglu. "Detection of Helicobacter pylori seropositivity in hyperemesis gravidarum and correlation with symptoms." *American Journal of Perinatology* 19 (Feb 2002): 87–92.

Furneaux, E.C., A.J. Langley-Evans, and S.C. Langley-Evans. "Nausea and vomiting of pregnancy: endocrine basis and contribution to pregnancy outcome." *Obstetrical and Gynecological Survey* 56 (Dec 2001): 775–82.

Jewell, D. "Nausea and vomiting in early pregnancy." *Clinical Evidence* 7 (2001): 1277–83.

Jewell, D., and G. Young. "Interventions for nausea and vomiting in early pregnancy" (Cochrane Review). In: *The Cochrane Library*, Issue 1, 2004. Chichester, UK: John Wiley & Sons, Ltd.

Knight, B., C. Mudge, S. Openshaw, A. White, and A. Hart. "Effect of acupuncture on nausea of pregnancy; a randomized, controlled trial." *Obstetrics and Gynecology* 97 (Feb 2001): 184–8.

Mazzotta, P., L.A. Magee, and G. Koren. "The association between abortion and nausea and vomiting of pregnancy." *Motherisk*. 2002. http://www.nvp-volumes.org/p2/.

Murphy, P.A. "Alternative therapies for nausea and vomiting of pregnancy." *Obstetrics and Gynecology* 91 (Jan 1998): 149–55.

Neutel, C.I. "Variation in rates of hospitalization for excessive vomiting in pregnancy by Bendectin/Diclectin use in Canada." *Motherisk*. 2000. http://www.nvp-volumes.org/p1_9.htm/.

Smith, C., C. Crowther, and J. Beilby. "Acupuncture to treat nausea and vomiting in early pregnancy: a randomized controlled trial." *Birth* 29 (March 2002): 1–9.

Vutyavanich, T., T. Kraisarin, and R-A. Ruangsri. "Ginger for nausea and vomiting in pregnancy: randomized, double-masked, placebo-controlled trial." *Obstetrics and Gynecology* 97 (April 2001): 577–82.

Wiegel, R.M. "Nausea and vomiting in pregnancy and pregnancy outcome: an epidemiological overview." *Motherisk*. 2000. http://www.nvp-volumes.org/pl_7.htm/.

CHAPTER SIX

Grunebaum, Dr. Amos. "Ask Our Experts." *WebMD Corporation*. 2001. http://www.content.health.msn.com/question_and_answer/article/3608.705/.

"A Healthy Pregnancy." *Bandolier EXTRA*. http://www.ebandolier.com/.

"Caffeine." *Center for the Evolution of Risks to Human Reproduction*. May 17, 2002. http://www.cerhr.niehs.nih.gov/genpub/topics/caffeine-ccae.html/.

"Caffeine and Health." *Bandolier Library*. December 1998. http://www.jr2.ox.ac.uk/Band58/b58-4/html#Heading2/.

"Caffeine and Pregnancy." *Organization of Teratology Information Services*. December 2001. http://www.OTISpregnancy.org/.

"Consumer Advisory Center for Food Safety and Applied Nutrition." *U.S. Food and Drug Administration*. March 2001.

"Department of Health and Human Services FDA and FSIS Issue Health Advisory About Listeria." *FDA News. U.S. Food and Drug Administration*. September 13, 2001.

Duffy, V.B., and G.H. Anderson. "Use of nutritive and nonnutritive sweeteners—position of ADA." *Journal of the American Diet Association* 98 (May 1998): 580–7.

Duley, L., and D. Smart-Henderson. "Reduced salt intake compared to normal dietary salt, or high intake, in pregnancy" (Cochrane Review). In: *The Cochrane Library*, Issue 3, 2002. Oxford, UK: Update Software, Ltd.

Easmon, C. "Prevention of malaria." NetDoctor.Co.UK. October 21, 2002. http://www.netdoctor.co.uk/diseases/facts/malaria.htm/.

Frank, L., A. Marian, M. Visser, E. Weinberg, and P.C. Potter. Exposure to peanuts *in utero* and in infancy and the development of sensitization to peanut allergens in young children. *Pediatric Allergy and Immunology* 10 (Feb 1999): 27–32.

"Go Ask Alice!: Okay to eat sushi and yogurt during pregnancy?" *Columbia University's Health Question & Answer Internet Service.* Nov 2000. http://www.goaskalice.columbia.edu/1464.html/.

Goldberg, G.R., A.M. Prentice, W.A. Coward, H.L. Davies, P.R. Murgatroyd, C. Wensing, A.E. Black, M. Harding, and M. Sawyer. "Longitudinal assessment of energy expenditure in pregnancy by the doubly labeled water method." *American Journal of Clinical Nutrition* 57 (April 1993): 494–505.

"Iron Content of Common Foods—Health File #68D." British Columbia Ministry of Health. February 2002. www.hlth.gov.bc.ca/hlthfile/hfile68d.html/.

"Listeriosis and Pregnancy." *Organization of Teratology Information Services.* December 2001. http://www.otispregnancy.org/.

McAnulty, P.A., M.J. Collier, J. Enticott, J.M. Tesh, D.A. Mayhew, C.P. Comer, J.J. Hjelle, and F.N. Kotsonis. "Absence of developmental effects in CF-1 mice exposed to aspartame in utero." *Fundamentals and Applied Toxicology* 13 (August 1989): 296–302.

"Mercury Levels in Seafood Species." *U.S. Food and Drug Administration Center for Food Safety and Applied Nutrition Office of Seafood,* May 2001.

"Multistate Outbreak of Listeriosis—United States." *MMWR Morbidity and Mortality Weekly Report* 49. December 22, 2000.

Nurminen, T. "Maternal pesticide exposure and pregnancy outcome." *Journal of Occupational and Environmental Medicine* 37 (August 1995): 935–40.

"Quantitative Assessment of the Relative Risk to Public Health from Foodborne *Listeria monocytogenes* Among Selected Categories for Ready-to-Eat Foods." *Center for Food Safety and Applied Nutrition. FDA. US DHHS.* September 2003.

Siegman-Igra, Y., R. Levin, M. Weinberger, Y. Golan, D. Schwartz, Z. Samra, H. Konigsberger, A. Yinnon, G. Rahav, N. Keller, N. Bisharat, J. Karpuch, R. Finkelstein, M. Alkan, Z. Landau, J. Novikov, D. Hassin, C. Ruddnick, R. Kitzes, S. Ovadia, Z. Shimoni, R. Lang, and T. Shohat. "Listeria monocytogenes infection in Israel and review of cases worldwide." *Emerging Infectious Diseases* 8 (March 2002): 305–10.

Sturtevant, F.M. "Use of aspartame in pregnancy." *International Journal of Fertility* 30 (1985): 85–7.

"Toxoplasmosis and Pregnancy." *Organization of Teratology Information Services*. August 1997. http://www.otispregnancy.org/.

van den Berg, H., K.F. Hulshof, and J.P. Deslypere. "Evaluation of the effect of the use of vitamin supplements on vitamin A intake among (potentially) pregnant women in relation to the consumption of liver and liver products." *European Journal of Obstetrics and Gynecology and Reproductive Biology* 66 (May 1996): 17–21.

Valtin, H. "'Drink at least eight glasses of water a day.' Really? Is there scientific evidence of '8 x 8'?" *American Journal of Physiol Regu Physiol* (Aug 2002).

CHAPTER SEVEN

Abalos, E., L. Duley, D.W. Steyn, and D.J. Henderson-Smart. "Antihypertensive drug therapy for mild to moderate hypertension during pregnancy" (Cochrane Review). In: *The Cochrane Library,* Issue 3, 2002. Oxford, UK: Update Software, Ltd.

Bauters, T.G., M.A. Dhont, M.I. Temmerman, and H.J. Nelis. "Prevalence of vulvovaginal candidiasis and susceptibility to fluconazole in women." *American Journal of Obstetrics and Gynecology* 187 (Sep 2002): 569–74.

"Chicken Pox and Pregnancy." *Organization of Teratology Information Services*. August 1997. http://www.otispregnancy.org/.

"Chickenpox in Pregnancy—Small but Real Risk." *Motherisk*. Feb 2001. http://www.motherisk.org/diseases/risktext.php3/.

Cook, A.J., R.E. Gilbert, W. Buffolano, J. Zufferey, E. Petersen, P.A. Jenum, W. Foulon, A.E. Semprini, and D.T. Dunn on behalf of the European Research Network on Congenital Toxoplasmosis. "Sources of toxoplasma infection in pregnant women: European multicenter case-control study." *BMJ* 321 (July 15 2000): 142–7.

"Critical review of the effects of prior and subsequent pregnancy on the prognosis of young women with breast cancer." *Motherisk*. June 2001. http://www.motherisk.org/cancer/critical.php3/.

"Cytomegalovirus and Pregnancy." *Organization of Teratology Information Services*. December 2001. http://www.otispregnancy.org/.

"Cytomegalovirus (CMV) Infection." *National Center for Infectious Diseases*. CDC. http://www.cdc.gov/ncidod/diseases/cmv.htm/.

Dwyer, P.L., and M. O'Reilly. "Recurrent urinary tract infection in the female." *Current Opinion in Obstetrics and Gynecology* 14 (2002): 537–43.

"Fifth Disease and Pregnancy." *Organization of Teratology Information Services.* January 2002. http://www.otispregnancy.org/.

"Hyperthermia and Pregnancy." *Organization of Teratology Information Services.* May 1998. http://www.otispregnancy.org/.

"Influenza and the Vaccine During Pregnancy." *Organization of Teratology Information Services.* November 2000. http://www.otispregnancy.org/.

Inman, W., G. Pearce, and L. Wilton. "Safety of fluconazole in the treatment of vaginal candidiasis. A prescription-event monitoring study, with special reference to the outcome of pregnancy." *European Journal of Clinical Pharmacology* 46 (1994): 115–8.

Inocencion, G., R. Loebstein, A. Lalkin, R. Geist, M. Petric, and G. Koren. "Managing exposure to chickenpox during pregnancy." *Motherisk.* April 1998. http://www.motherisk.org/updates/april98.php3/.

Jones, J.L., A. Lopez, M. Wilson, J. Schulkin, and R. Gibbs. "Congenital toxoplasmosis: a review." *Obstetrical and Gynecological Survey* 56 (May 2001): 296–305.

Koren, G. "Varicella virus vaccine before pregnancy." *Motherisk.* October 2000. http://www.motherisk.org/updates/oct00.php3/.

Lalkim, A., R. Loebstein, A. Addis, and G. Koren. "Therapeutic approach to hypertension during pregnancy." *Motherisk.* June 1998. http://www.motherisk.org/updates/jun98.php3/.

Magee, L.A., and L. Duley. "Oral beta-blockers for mild to moderate hypertension during pregnancy" (Cochrane Review). In: *The Cochrane Library,* Issue 3, 2002. Chichester, UK: John Wiley & Sons, Ltd.

Mankuta, D., B. Bar-Oz, and G. Koren. "Erythema infectiosum (Fifth disease) and pregnancy." *Motherisk.* March 1999. http://www.motherisk.org/updates/mar99.php3/.

Millar, L.K., L. Debuque, and D.A. Wing. "Uterine contraction frequency during treatment of pyelonephritis in pregnancy and subsequent risk of preterm birth." *Journal of Perinatal Medicine* 31 (2003): 41–46.

Nulman, I., D. Laslo, and G. Koren. "Treatment of epilepsy in pregnancy." *Drugs* 57 (April 1999): 535–44.

"Paxil (paroxetine) and Pregnancy." *Organization of Teratology Information Services.* November 2000. http://www.otispregnancy.org/.

"Perinatal Viral and Parasitic Infections." *ACOG Practice Bulletin Number 20.* September 2000. Published by American College of Obstetricians & Gynecologists, Washington D.C.

"Phentermine and Pregnancy." *Organization of Teratology Information Services.* May 2000. http://www.otispregnancy.org/.

"Pregnancy and Breast Cancer." *Clinical Green Top Guideline No 12. Jan 2004. Scientific Advisory Committee of the Royal College of Obstetricians and Gynaecologists.* http://www.rcog.org.uk/guidelines.asp?PageID=106& GuidelineID=6/.

"Prozac (fluoxetine) and Pregnancy." *Organization of Teratology Information Services.* June 2001. http://www.otispregnancy.org/.

"Retin-A and Pregnancy." *Organization of Teratology Information Services.* November 2000. http://www.otispregnancy.org/.

Sorensen, H.T., G.L. Nielsen, C. Olesen, H. Larsen, F.H. Steffensen, H.C. Schonheyder, J. Olsen, and A.E. Czeizel. "Risk of malformations and other outcomes in children exposed to fluconazole in utero." *British Journal of Clinical Pharmacology* 48 (1999): 234–8.

"St. John's Wort (Hypericum perforatum) and Pregnancy." *Organization of Teratology Information Services.* October 2000. http://www.otispregnancy.org/.

"Tegretol (carbamazepine) and Pregnancy." *Organization of Teratology Information Services.* August 2001. http://www.otispregnancy.org/.

"Tetracycline and Pregnancy." *Organization of Teratology Information Services.* November 2000. http://www.otispregnancy.org/.

Theis, J.G.W. "Acetysalicylic acid (ASA) and nonsteroidal anti-inflammatory drugs (NSAIDs) during pregnancy. Are they safe?" *Motherisk.* December 1996. http://www.motherisk.org/updates/dec96.php3/.

Young, G.L., and D. Jewell. "Antihistamines versus aspirin for itching in late pregnancy" (Cochrane Review). In: *The Cochrane Library,* Issue 3, 2002. Oxford, UK: Update Software, Ltd.

Young, G.L., and D. Jewell. "Topical treatment for vaginal candidiasis (thrush) in pregnancy." (Cochrane Review). In: *The Cochrane Library,* Issue 1, 2004, Chichester, UK: John Wiley & Sons, Ltd.

CHAPTER EIGHT

Addis, A., M.E. Moretti, F. Ahmed Syed, T.R. Einarson, and G. Koren. "Fetal effects of cocaine: an updated meta-analysis." *Reproductive Toxicology* 15 (Jul–Aug 2001): 341–69.

Taylor, D.J. "Alcohol Consumption in Pregnancy." Clinical Green Top Guidelines. *Guidelines and Audit Sub-Committee of the Royal College of Obstetricians and Gynaecologists.* Dec 1999. http://www.rcog.org.uk/print.asp?PageID=106&Type=guidelines&GuidelineID=1/.

Center for Reproductive Law & Policy. *Punishing Women for Their Behavior During Pregnancy: An Approach that Undermines Women's Health and Children's Interests.* Part 1. New York: Center for Reproductive Law & Policy, 1996.

"Cocaine and Pregnancy." *Organization of Teratology Information Services.* August 2001. http://www.otispregnancy.org/.

Conde-Agudelo, A., F. Althabe, J.M. Belizan, and A.C. Kafury-Goeta. "Cigarette smoking during pregnancy and risk of preeclampsia: a systematic review." *American Journal of Obstetrics and Gynecology* 181 (Oct 1999): 1026–35.

"The Fetus as a Passive Smoker." *Motherisk.* March 2001. http://www.motherisk.org/drugs/smoktext.php3/.

Frank, D.A., M. Augustyn, W.G. Knight, T. Pell, and B. Zuckerman. "Growth, development, and behavior in early childhood following prenatal cocaine exposure: a systematic review." *Journal of the American Medical Association* 285 (March 2001): 1613–25.

Fried, P.A., and A.M. Smith. "A literature review of the consequences of prenatal marijuana exposure: An emerging theme of a deficiency in aspects of executive function." *Neurotoxicology and Teratology* 23 (Jan–Feb 2001): 1–11.

Hall, W., and D. MacPhee. "Cannabis use and cancer." *Addiction* 97 (Mar 2002): 243–7.

Hughes, E.G., and B.G. Brennan. "Does cigarette smoking impair natural or assisted fecundity?" *Fertility and Sterility* 66 (November 1996): 679–89.

Koren, G. "Alcohol consumption in early pregnancy." *Motherisk.* Nov 1996. http://www.motherisk.org/updates/nov96.php3/.

Polygenis, D., S. Wharton, C. Malmberg, N. Sherman, D. Kennedy, G. Koren, and T.R. Einarson. "Moderate alcohol consumption during pregnancy and the incidence of fetal malformations: a meta-analysis." *Neurotoxicology and Teratology* 20 (Jan–Feb 1998): 61–7.

Scalera, A., and G. Koren. "Rationale for treating pregnant smokers with nicotine patches." *Motherisk.* August 1998. http://www.motherisk.org/updates/aug98.php3/.

Shah, N.R., and M.B. Bracken. "A systematic review and meta-analysis of prospective studies on the association between maternal cigarette smoking and preterm delivery." *American Journal of Obstetrics and Gynecology* 182 (Feb 2000): 465–72.

"Smoking during pregnancy and risk of oral clefts." *Bandolier Library.* Aug 2002. http://www.jr2.ox.ac.uk/bandolier/booth/hliving/Smpreclf.html/.

Thorogood, M., M. Hillsdon, and C. Summerbelt. "Cardiovascular disorders— changing behavior." *Clinical Evidence.* BMJ Publishing Group, London (2003): 17–18.

CHAPTER NINE

"Exercise during pregnancy and the postpartum period." *ACOG. Technical Bulletin.* Number 267, Jan 2002. Published by American College of Obstetricians & Gynecologists, Washington, D.C.

"Aerobic exercise for women during pregnancy" (Cochrane Review) In: *The Cochrane Library,* Issue 3, 2002. Oxford, UK: Update Software, Ltd.

Artal, R., and R. Wisell, eds. *Exercise in Pregnancy.* Baltimore, MD: Williams & Wilkins, 1986.

Boissonnault, J.S., and M.J. Blaschak. "Incidence of diastasis recti abdominis during the childbearing year." *Physical Therapy* 68 (Jul 1988): 1082–6.

Clapp, J.F., and S. Dickstein. "Endurance exercise and pregnancy outcome." *Medicine and Science in Sports and Exercise* 16 (Dec 1984): 556–62.

Cook, A.J., R.E. Gilbert, W. Buffolano, J. Zufferey, E. Petersen, P.A. Jenum, W. Fouon, A.E. Semprini, D.T. Dunn, and R. Holliman. "Sources of toxoplasma infection in pregnant women: European multicentre case-control study." *BMJ* 321 (Jul 15 2000): 142–7.

Gardella, J.R., and J.A. Hill. "Environmental toxins associated with recurrent pregnancy loss." *Seminars in Reproductive Medicine* 18 (2000): 407–24.

Hsia, M., and S. Jones. "Natural resolution of rectus abdominis diastasis. Two single case studies." *Australian Journal of Physiotherapy* 46 (2000): 301–7.

Marnach, M.L., K.D. Ramin, P.S. Ramsey, S.W. Song, J.J. Stensland, and K.N. An. "Characterization of the relationship between joint laxity and maternal hormones in pregnancy." *Obstetrics and Gynecology* 101 (Feb 2003): 331–5.

Papiernik, E., and M. Kaminski. "Multifactorial study of the risk of prematurity at 32 weeks of gestation." *Journal of Perinatal Medicine* 2 (1974): 30–6.

Pergament, E., A. Schechtman, and A. Rochanayon. "Hyperthermia and pregnancy." Illinois Teratogen Information Service. June 1997. http://www.fetal-exposure.nwu.edu/HYPERTH.html/.

Sasaki, J., A. Yamaguchi, Y. Nabeshima, S. Shigemitsu, N. Mesaki, and T. Kubo. "Exercise at high temperature causes maternal hyperthermia and fetal anomalies in rats." *Teratology* 51 (Apr 1995): 233–6.

"Spas, Hot Tubs, and Whirlpools." CPSC Document #5112. *Consumer Product Safety Commission.* October 18, 2003. http://www.cpsc.gov/cpscpub/pubs/5112.html/.

Dye, T.D., and D. Oldenettel. "Physical activity and the risk of preterm labor: an epidemiological review and synethesis of recent literature." Seminars in Perinatology 20 (Aug. 1996): 334–9.

Kramer, M.S. "Aerobic exercise for women during pregnancy (Cochrane Review). In: *The Cochrane Library,* Issue 3, 2002. Oxford: Update Software.

CHAPTER TEN

Harvey, M.A. "Pelvic floor exercises during and after pregnancy: a systematic review of their role in preventing pelvic floor dysfunction." *Journal of Obstetrics and Gynaecology Canada* 25 (June 2003): 487–98.

Ruigomez, A., L.A. Garcia Rodriguez, C. Cattaruzzi, M.G. Troncon, L. Agostinis, M.A. Wallander, and S. Johansson. "Use of cimetidine, omeprazole, and ranitidine in pregnant women and pregnancy outcomes." *American Journal of Epidemiology* 150 (Sept 1 1999): 476–81.

Thorp, J.M. Jr., P.A. Norton, L.L. Wall, J.A. Kuller, B. Eucker, and E. Wells. "Urinary incontinence in pregnancy and the puerperium: a prospective study." *American Journal of Obstetrics and Gynecology* 181 (Aug. 1999): 266–73.

Young, G.L., and D. Jewell. "Interventions for leg cramps in pregnancy" (Cochrane Review). In: *The Cochrane Library,* Issue 3, 2002. Oxford, UK: Update Software, Ltd.

Jewell, D. and G.L. Young. "Interventions for treating constipation in pregnancy (Cochrane Review). In: *The Cochrane Library,* Issue 3, 2002. Oxford OK: Update Software, Ltd.

Young, G.L., and D. Jewell. "Interventions for varicosities and leg oedema in pregnancy" (Cochrane Review). In: *The Cochrane Library,* Issue 3, 2002. Oxford, UK: Update Software, Ltd.

CHAPTER ELEVEN

"Advice on Preventing Deep Vein Thrombosis for Pregnant Women Travelling by Air." *Scientific Advisory Committee Opinion Paper. Scientific Advisory Committee of the Royal College of Obstetricians and Gynaecologists.* October 1, 2001.

"Air travel during pregnancy." ACOG Committee on Obstetric Practice Opinion Number 264. *Obstetrics and Gynecology* 98 (Dec 2001): 1187–8.

Barish, R.J. "In-flight radiation: counseling patients about risk." *Journal of the American Board of Family Practice* 12 (May–Jun 2000): 195–9.

Johnson, H.C., and D.W. Pring. "Car seatbelts in pregnancy: the practice and knowledge of pregnant women remain causes for concern." *British Journal of Obstetrics and Gynaecology* 107 (May 2000): 644–7.

Klinish, K.D., L.W. Schneider, J.L. Moore, and M.D. Pearlman. "Investigations of crashes involving pregnant occupants." *44th Annual Proceedings Association for the Advancement of Automotive Medicine.* October 20–24, 2000.

CHAPTER TWELVE

Bialobok, K.M., and M. Monga. "Fatigue and work in pregnancy." *Current Opinion in Obstetrics and Gynecology* 12 (Dec 2000): 497–500.

Clapp, J.F., III. "Pregnancy outcome: physical activities inside versus outside the workplace." *Seminars in Perinatology* 20 (Feb 1996): 70–6.

El Metwalli, A.G., A.M. Badawy, L.A. El-Baghdadi, and A. Wehady. "Occupational physical activity and pregnancy outcome." *European Journal of Obstetrics and Gynecology and Reproductive Biology* 100 (Dec 2001): 41–5.

CHAPTER THIRTEEN

"Adverse Pregnancy Outcome Associated with the Use of Visual Display Units." Clinical Green Top Guidelines. *Royal College of Obstetricians and Gynaecologists.* 2002. http://www.rcog.org/uk/guidelines.asp?PageID=106&GuidelineID=23/.

Bentur, Y., and G. Koren. "The three most common occupational exposures reported by pregnant women: an update." *American Journal of Obstetrics and Gynecology* 165 (1999): 429–37.

"From the Editors: Protecting Against Congenital Toxoplasmosis." *Eurosurveillance Weekly* 24. June 1999. http://www.eurosurv.org/1999/pfp/990610.pfp.html/.

Khattak, S., G. K-Moghtader, K. McMartin, M. Barrera, D. Kennedy, and G. Koren. "Pregnancy outcome following gestational exposure to organic solvents: a prospective controlled study." *Journal of the American Medical Association* 281 (1999): 1106–9.

McMartin, K.J., and G. Koren. "Exposure to organic solvents." *Motherisk.* July 1999. http://www.motherisk.org/updates/jul99.php3/.

"NPT-CERHR Report on the Potential Reproductive and Developmental Effects of Di-n-Butyl Phthalate (DBP)." *National Toxicology Program NTP*

Center for the Evaluation of Risks to Human Reproduction National Institute of Environmental Health Science. http://www.cerhr.niehs.nih.gov/.

Moienafshari, R., B. Bar-oz, G. Koren. "Occupational exposure to mercury." *Motherisk*. January 1999. http://www.motherisk.org/updates/jan99.php3/.

Whiting, P., M. McDonagh, and J. Kleijnen. "Association of Down's syndrome and water fluoride level: a systematic review of the evidence." *BMC Public Health* 1 (2001): 6.

CHAPTER FOURTEEN

Berkman, N.D., J.M. Thorp Jr., K.E. Hartmann, K.N. Lohn, A.E. Idicula, M. McPheeters, N.I. Gavin, T.S. Carey, S. Tolleson-Rinehart, A.M. Jackman, V. Hasselblad, and E.C. Puckett. "Management of Preterm Labor." *Evidence Report/Technology Assessment Number 18. AHRG Publication Number 01-E012*. Rockville, MD: Agency for Healthcare Research and Quality, 2000.

"Epidurals and labour." *Bandolier Library*. October 1999. http://www.jr2. ox.ac.uk/bandolier/band68/b68-7.html/.

Howell, C.J., T. Dean, L. Lucking, K. Dziedzic, P.W. Jones, and R.B. Johanson. "Randomised study of long term outcome after epidural versus non-epidural analgesia during labour." *BJM* 325 (2002): 357.

CHAPTER FIFTEEN

Bainbridge, J. "Choices after cesarean." *Birth* 29 (2002): 203–6.

Bernath, V. "Lavender oil for perineal healing following childbirth." Centre for Clinical Effectiveness. 2002. http://www.med.monash.edu.au/healthservices/cce/evidence/pdf/b/763.pdf/.

Gupta, J., and V.C. Nikodem. "Position for women during second stage of labour" (Cochrane Review). In: *The Cochrane Library*, Issue 3, 2002. Oxford, UK: Update Software, Ltd.

Hannah, M.E., W.J. Hannah, S.A. Hewson, E.D. Hodnett, S. Saigal, and A.R. Willan for the Term Breech Trial Collaborative Group. "Planned caesarean section versus planned vaginal birth for breech presentation at term: a randomised multicentre trial." *Lancet* 356 (2000): 1375–83.

Hannah, M.E., W.J. Hannah, E.D. Hodnett, B. Chalmers, R. Kung, A. Willan, K. Amankwah, M. Cheng, M. Helewa, S. Hewson, S. Saigal, H. Whyte and A. Gafni. "Outcomes at 3 months after planned cesarean vs planned vaginal delivery for breech presentation at term. The International Randomized

Term Breech Trial." *Journal of the American Medical Association* 287 (2002): 1822–31.

Hofmeyr, G.J., and R. Kulier. "Hands/knees posture in late pregnancy or labour for fetal malposition (lateral or posterior)" (Cochrane Review). In: *The Cochrane Library*, Issue 3, 2002. Oxford, UK: Update Software, Ltd.

Jackson, N. and S. Paterson-Brown. "Physical sequelae of caesarean section. Best practice & research." *Clinical Obstetrics and Gynaecology* 15 (Feb 2001): 49–61.

Johanson, R.B., and V. Menon. "Vacuum extraction versus forceps for assisted vaginal delivery" (Cochrane Review). In: *The Cochrane Library*, Issue 3, 2002. Oxford, UK: Update Software, Ltd.

"Management of Genital Herpes in Pregnancy." *Clinical Green Top Guidelines*. March 2002. http://www.rcog.org.uk/print.asp?PageID=106&Type=guidelines&Guideline/.

McMahon, M.J., E.R. Luther, W.A. Bowes Jr., and A.F. Olshan. "Comparison of a trial of labor with an elective second cesarean section." *New England Journal of Medicine* 335 (Sep 1996): 689–95.

Miksovsky, P., and W.J. Watson. "Obstetric vacuum extraction: stage of the art in the new millennium." *Obstetrical and Gynecological Survey* 56 (Nov 2001): 736–51.

"Mode of Term Singleton Breech Delivery." ACOG Committee Opinion. *The American College of Obstetricians and Gynecologists*. Washington, D.C. 2001.

Neri, I., M. Fazzio, S. Menghini, A. Volpe, and F. Facchinetti. "Non-stress test changes during acupuncture plus moxibustion on BL67 point in breech presentation." *Journal of the Society for Gynecologic Investigation* 9 (May–Jun 2002): 158–62.

Nikodem, V.C. "Immersion in water in pregnancy, labour and birth" (Cochrane Review). In: *The Cochrane Library*, Issue 1, 2004. Chichester, UK: John Wiley & Sons, Ltd.

Sanchez-Ramos, L., S. Bernstein, and A.M. Kaunitz. "Expectant management versus labor induction for suspected fetal macrosomia: a systematic review." *Obstetrics and Gynecology* 100 (Nov 2002): 997–1002.

Thompson, J.F., C.L. Roberts, M. Currie, and D.A. Ellwood. "Prevalence and persistence of health problems after childbirth: associations with parity and method of birth." *Birth* 29 (Jun 2002): 83–94.

Walker, R., D. Turnbull, and C. Wilkinson. "Strategies to address global cesarean section rates: a review of the evidence." *Birth* 29 (Mar 2002): 28–39.

CHAPTER SIXTEEN

"Breastfeeding and the Use of Human Milk (RE9729)." *American Academy of Pediatrics.* Volume 100, Number 6. (December 1997): 1035–9.

Barbosa-Cesnik, C., K. Schwartz, and B. Foxman. "Lactation mastitis." *Journal of the American Medical Association* 289 (Apr 2 2003): 1609–12.

"Breastfeeding: Maternal and Infant Aspects." *ACOG Educational Bulletin Number 258.* July 2000. American College of Obstetricians & Gynecologists, Washington, D.C.

Hender, K. "Infant formula compared to breast milk for the prevention of allergies in neonates." *Centre for Clinical Effectiveness.* 2001. http://www.med.monash.edu.au/healthservices/cce/.

Ito, S. "Drug therapy for breast-feeding women." *New England Journal of Medicine* 343 (Jul 13 2000): 118–26.

Koletzko, B., and F. Lehner. "Beer and breastfeeding." *Advances in Experimental Medicine and Biology* 478 (2000): 23–8.

Little, R.E., K. Northstone, J. Golding, and ALSPAC Study Team. "Alcohol, breastfeeding, and development at 18 months." *Pediatrics* 109 (May 2002): E72–2.

Mennella, J.A., and G.K. Beauchamp. "The transfer of alcohol to human milk. Effects on flavor and the infant's behavior." *New England Journal of Medicine* 325 (Oct 1991): 981–5.

Moretti, M.E., A. Lee, and S. Ito. "Which drugs are contraindicated during breastfeeding? Practice Guidelines." *Motherisk.* September 2000. http://www.motherisk.org/updates/sept00.php3/.

The World Health Organization Multinational Study of Breast-feeding and Lactational Amenorrhea III. "Pregnancy during breast-feeding." *Fertility and Sterility* 72 (Sep 1999): 431–40.

CHAPTER SEVENTEEN

Abraham, S., A. Child, J. Ferry, J. Vizzard, and M. Mira. "Recovery after childbirth: a preliminary prospective study." *The Medical Journal of Australia* 152 (Jan 1 1990): 9–12.

"Circumcision." The American College of Obstetricians and Gynecologists. Number 260. October 2001. ACOG. Washington, D.C.

Kettle, C., and R.B. Johanson. "Continuous versus interrupted sutures for perineal repair" (Cochrane Review). In: *The Cochrane Library,* Issue 1, 2004. Chichester, UK: John Wiley & Sons, Ltd.

Dixon, M., N. Booth, and R. Powell. "Sex and relationships following child-birth: a first report from general practice of 131 couples." *British Journal of General Practice* 50 (Mar 2000): 223–4.

Eastham, J.H. "Postpartum alopecia." *Annals of Pharmacotherapy* 35 (Feb 2001): 255–8.

Gjerdingen, D. "Expectant parents' anticipated changes in workload after the birth of their first child." *Journal of Family Practice* 49 (Nov 2000): 993–7.

Gjerdingen, D.K., D.G. Froberg, K.M. Chaloner, and P.M. McGovern. "Changes in women's physical health during the first postpartum year." *Archives of Family Medicine* 2 (Mar 1993): 277–83.

Gold, L.H. "Postpartum disorders in primary care: diagnosis and treatment." *Primary Care* 29 (Mar 2002): 27–41.

Grant, A., B. Gordon, C. Mackrodat, E. Fern, A. Truesdale, and S. Ayers. "The Ipswich childbirth study: one year follow up of alternative methods used in perineal repair." *BJOG* 108 (Jan 2001): 34–40.

Groutz, A. G. Fait, J.B. Lessing, M.P. David, I. Wolman, A. Jaff, and D. Gordon. "Incidence and obstetric risk factors of postpartum anal incontinence." *Scandinavian Journal of Gastroenterology* 34 (Mar 1999): 315–8.

Hay-Smith, E.J. "Therapeutic ultrasound for postpartum perineal pain and dyspareunia." (Cochrane Review) In: The Cochrane Library Issue 1, 2004. Chichester, UK: John Wiley & Sons, Ltd.

"Healthy Post-Natal Care." *Bandolier Extra*. December 2001. http://www. ebandolier.com/.

Josefsson, A., G. Berg, C. Nordin, and G. Sydsjo. "Prevalence of depressive symptoms in late pregnancy and postpartum." *Acta Obstetricia et Gynecologica Scandinavica* 80 (Mar 2001): 251–5.

Killien, M.G. "Postpartum return to work: mothering stress, anxiety, and gratification." *Canadian Journal of Nursing Research* 30 (Fall 1998): 53–66.

Lee, K.A., and M.E. Zaffke. "Longitudinal changes in fatigue and energy during pregnancy and the postpartum period." *Journal of Obstetric, Gynecologic, and Neonatal Nursing* 28 (Mar 1999): 183–91.

MacArthur, C., D.E. Bick, and M.R. Keighley. "Faecal incontinence after childbirth." *British Journal of Obstetrics and Gynaecology* 104 (Jan 1997): 46–50.

McGovern, P., B. Dowd, D. Gjerdingen, I. Moscovice, L. Kochevar, and W. Lohman. "Time off work and the postpartum health of employed women." *Medical Care* 35 (May 1997): 507–21.

Pregazzi, R., A. Sartore, P. Bortoli, E. Grimaldi, G. Ricci, and S. Guaschino. "Immediate postpartum perineal examination as a predictor of puerperal pelvic floor dysfunction." *Obstetrics and Gynecology* 99 (Apr 2002): 581–4.

Pregazzi, R. A. Sartore, L. Troiano, E. Grimaldi, P. Bortoli, S. Siracusano, and S. Guaischino. "Postpartum urinary symptoms: prevalence and risk factors." *European Journal of Obstetrics and Gynecology and Reproductive Biology* 103 (Jul 10 2002):179–182.

Scott, K.D., P.H. Klaus, and M.H. Klaus. "The obstetrical and postpartum benefits of continuous support during childbirth." *Womens Health and Gender-Based Medicine* 8 (Dec 1999): 1257–64.

Signorello, L.B., B.L. Harlow, A.K. Chekos, and J.T. Repke. "Postpartum sexual functioning and the relationship to perineal trauma: a retrospective cohort study of primiparous women." *American Journal of Obstetrics and Gynecology* 184 (Apr 2001): 881–8.

Stamp, G. G. Kruzins, and C. Crowther. "Perineal massage in labour and prevention of perineal trauma: randomised controlled trial." *BMJ* 322 (May 26 2001): 1277–80.

Kettle, C., and R.B. Johanson. "Synthetic versus catgut suture material for perineal repair" (Cochrane Review). In: *The Cochrane Library*, Issue 1, 2004. Chichester, UK: John Wiley & Sons, Ltd.

Thompson, J.F., C.L. Roberts, M. Currie, and D.A. Ellwood. "Prevalence and persistence of health problems after childbirth: Associations with parity and method of birth." *Birth* 29 (Jun 2002): 83–94.

Von Sydow, K. "Sexuality during pregnancy and after childbirth: a metacontent analysis of 59 studies." *Journal of Psychosomatic Research* 47 (Jul 1999): 27–49.

Willis, A., A. Fardi, S. Schelzig, F. Hoelzl, R. Kasperk, W. Rath, and V. Schumpelick. "Childbirth and incontinence: a prospective study on anal sphincter morphology and function before and early after vaginal delivery." *Langenbecks Archives of Surgery* 387 (Jun 2002): 101–7.

International Labour Organization, Maternity Leave in Selected Countries, Geneva, 1998. http://www.ilo.org.

Acknowledgments

Writing this book would have been impossible if not for the help and guidance of many people. Nancy Crossman devoted her time and energy over several years to help me focus and define my original concept for this book. Sheila Curry Oakes at Perigee Books saw the fruits of these efforts, and helped turn a vision into a reality. Catherine Musicant, Nina Koh, Julie Macht, and Janet Eisenberg read drafts and gave ideas about how to improve the manuscript; these suggestions improved the book in so many ways. Thanks also to Kim Mowrey and Lisa Kaspin for transcription and editing help.

Finally, my wife Donna read innumerable early versions and provided countless helpful suggestions. She is the one person without whose help this book would certainly never have been written.

Index

About the Author

Michael S. Broder, MD, has focused much of his career on improving women's health. Dr. Broder graduated cum laude from Harvard University. He completed medical school at Case Western Reserve University and did his residency training at the UCLA School of Medicine. He has been on the faculty of the Ob-Gyn department at UCLA since 1996. In addition to being a board certified Obstetrician-Gynecologist, he has written extensively on a variety of subjects, including the overuse of hysterectomy, new treatments for uterine fibroids, and the quality of surgical care in the United States. Dr. Broder, along with Dr. Scott Goodwin, has written a book on treatments for uterine fibroids, called *What Your Doctor May Not Tell You About Fibroids*. His research has been discussed in numerous newspapers, magazines, and television shows, including the *Los Angeles Times, Health, Prevention,* and *20/20*. Dr. Broder is currently working on a third book. He lives in Beverly Hills with his wife and three children.